Things a
Lady
Would Like to
Know
Concerning
Health & Beauty

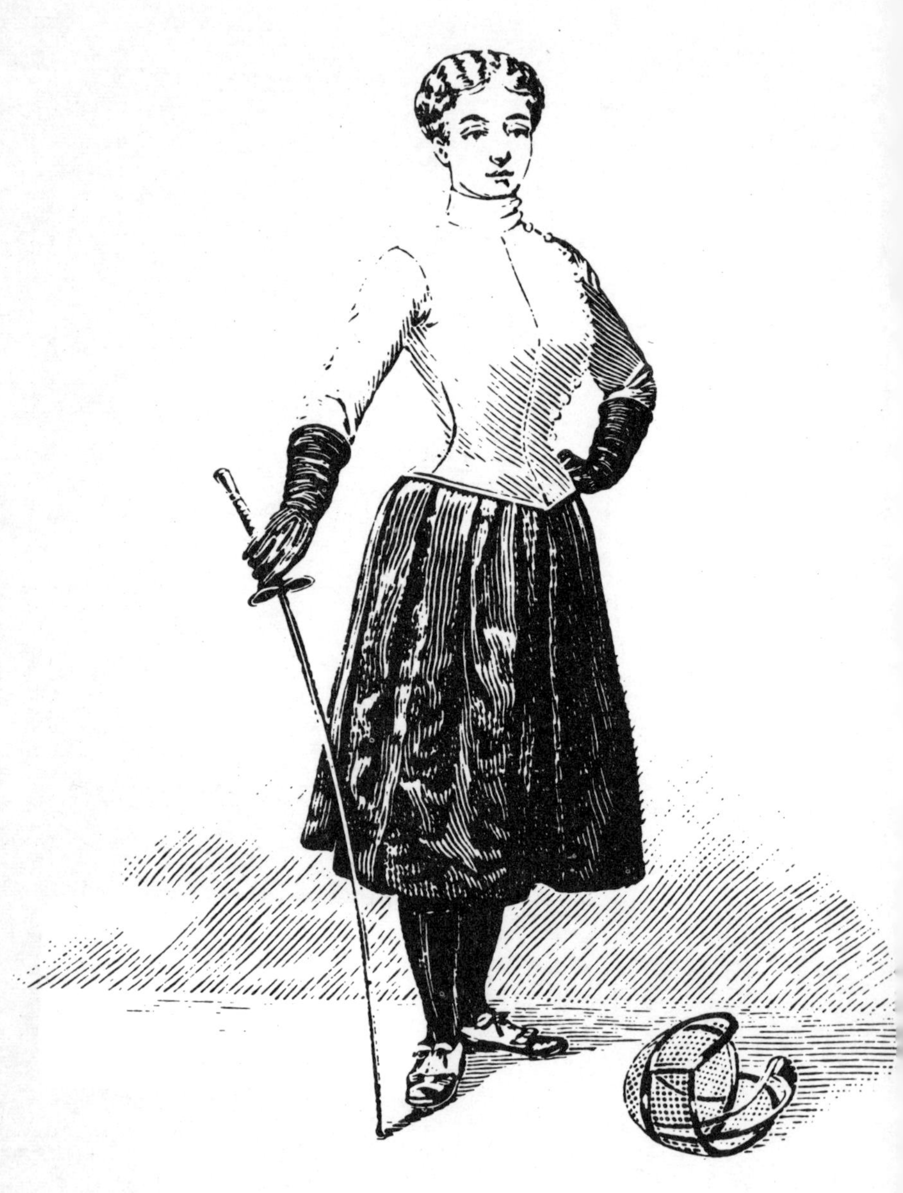

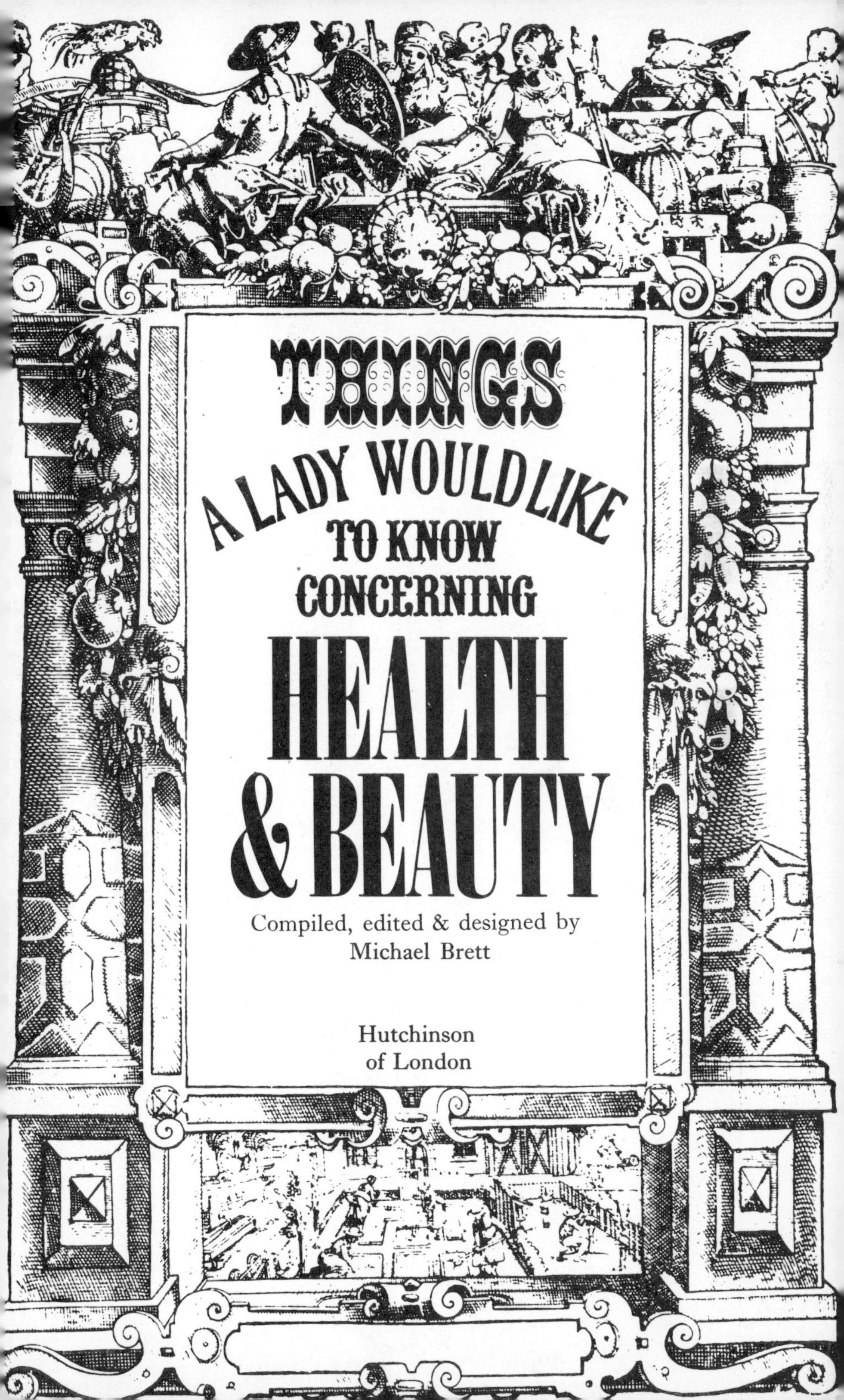

THINGS
A LADY WOULD LIKE TO KNOW
CONCERNING
HEALTH & BEAUTY

Compiled, edited & designed by
Michael Brett

Hutchinson
of London

HUTCHINSON & CO (*Publishers*) LTD
178–202 Great Portland Street, London, W.1.
London Melbourne Sydney
Auckland Johannesburg Cape Town
and agencies throughout the world

This selection
first published 1970

© This selection
Michael Brett 1970

Printed in Great Britain by offset litho
at Taylor Garnett Evans & Co. Ltd.
Watford, Herts, on Evensyde white offset,
set in Monotype Imprint.
Bound by Wm. Brendon & Son Ltd., Tiptree, Essex.
ISBN 0 09 104331 X

CONTENTS

To my wife
for all her
help and
patience

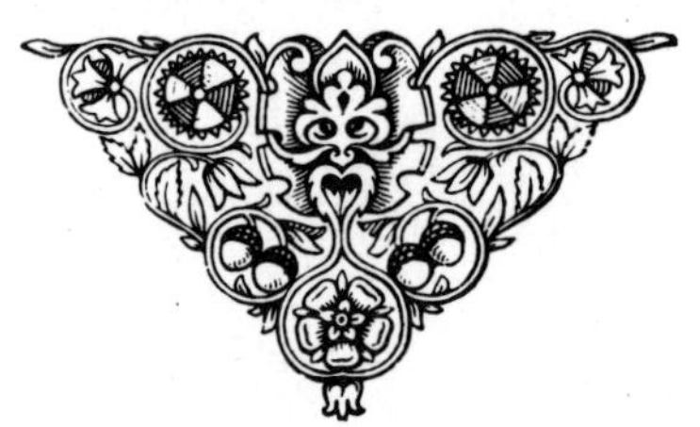

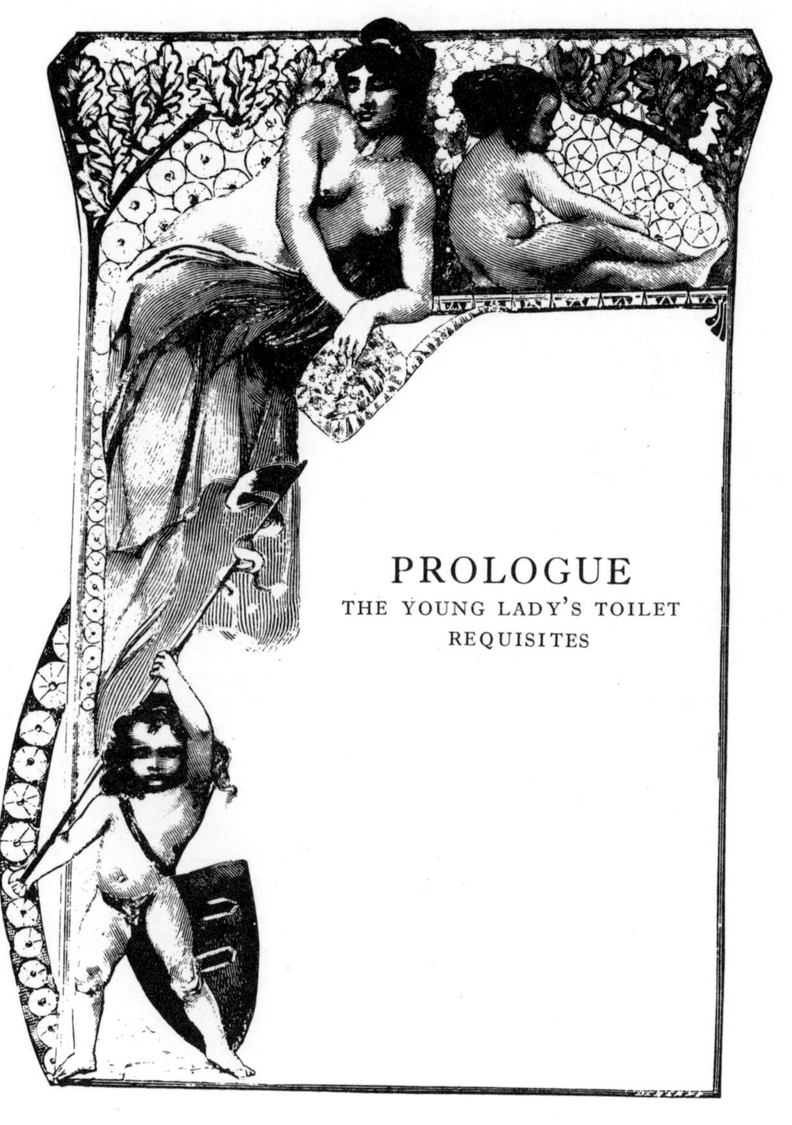

PROLOGUE
THE YOUNG LADY'S TOILET
REQUISITES

PROLOGUE

THE YOUNG LADY'S TOILET REQUISITES

The Enchanted Mirror—Self Knowledge
This curious glass will bring your faults to light
And make your virtues shine both strong and bright

Wash to Smooth Wrinkles—Contentment
A daily portion of this essence use
'Twill smooth the brow, and tranquility infuse.

Fine Lipsalve—Truth
Use daily for your lips this precious dye,
They'll redden, and breathe sweet melody.

Mixture for the Voice—Prayer
At morning, noon, and night this mixture take,
Your tones, improved, will richer music make.

Best Eye-Water—Compassion

These drops will add great lustre to the eye;
When more you need, the poor will you supply.

Solution to prevent Eruptions—Wisdom
It calms the temper, beautifies the face,
And gives to woman dignity and grace.

Matchless Pair of Ear-rings—Attention and Obedience
With these clear drops appended to the ear,
Attentive lessons you will gladly hear.

Indispensable Pair of Bracelets—Neatness and Industry
Clasp them on carefully each day you live,
To good designs they efficacy give.

An Elastic Girdle—Patience
The more you use the brighter it will grow,
Though its least merit its external show.

Ring of Tried Gold—Principle
Yield not this golden bracelet while you live,
" 'Twill sin restrain, and peace of conscience give".

Necklace of Purest Pearl—Resignation
This ornament embellishes the fair,
And teaches all the ills of life to bear.

Diamond Breast-pin—Love
Adorn your bosom with this precious pin,
It shines without, and warms the heart within.

A Graceful Bandeau—Politeness
The forehead neatly circled with this band,
Will admiration and respect command.

A Precious Diadem—Piety
Whoe'er this precious diadem shall own,
Secures herself an everlasting crown.

Universal Beautifier—Good Temper
With this choice liquid gently touch the mouth,
It spreads o'er all the face the charms of youth.

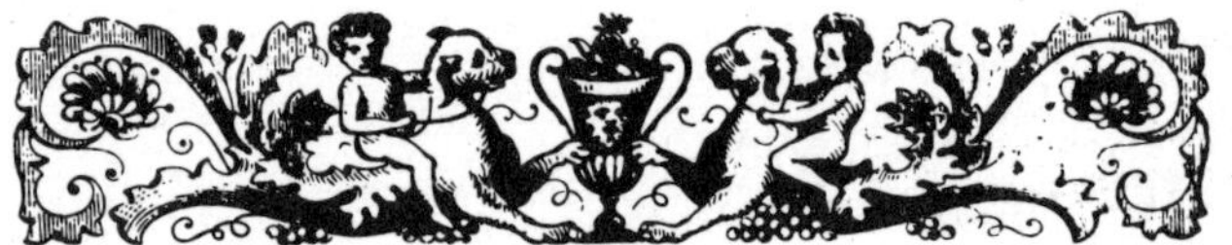

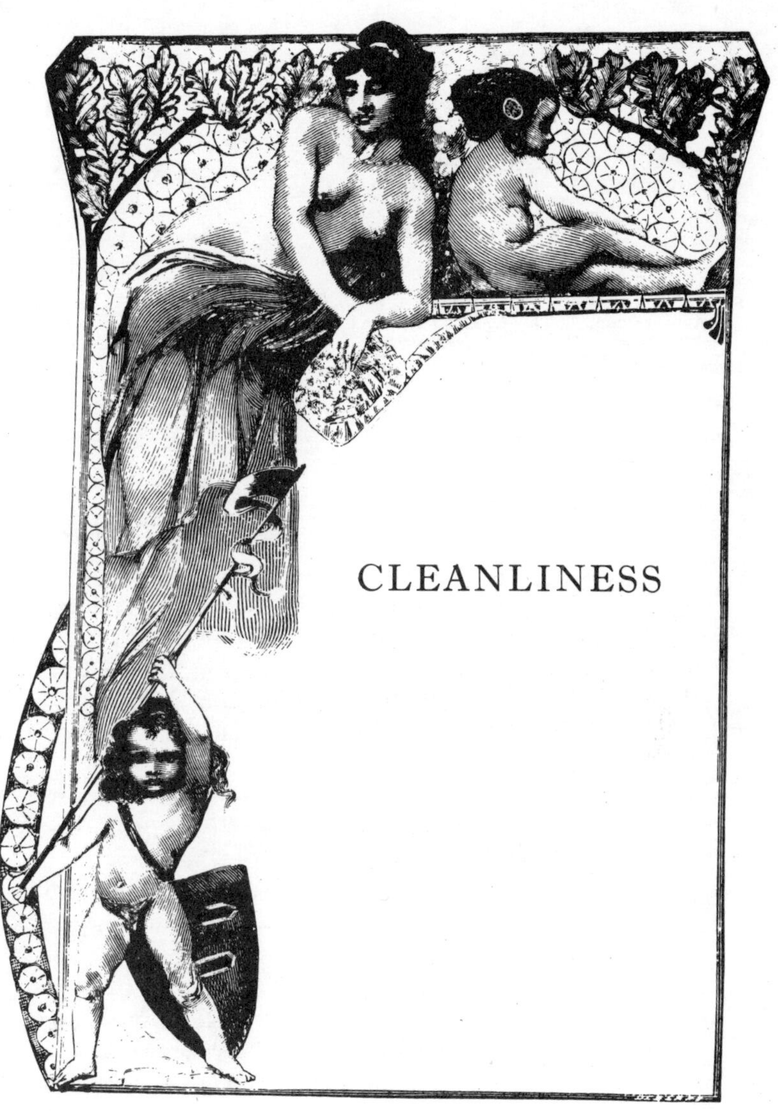

CLEANLINESS

CLEANLINESS

HE want of cleanliness is a fault which admits of no excuse. Where water can be had for nothing, it is surely in the power of every person to be clean. The discharge from our bodies by perspiration renders frequent changes of apparel necessary.

Change of apparel greatly promotes the secretion from the skin, so necessary to health.

When that matter which ought to be carried off by perspiration is either retained in the body, or reabsorbed in dirty clothes, it is apt to occasion fevers and other diseases.

Most diseases of the skin proceed from want of cleanliness. These indeed may be caught by infection, but they will seldom continue long where cleanliness prevails.

To the same cause must we impute the various kinds

of vermin that infest the human body, houses, &c. These may generally be banished by cleanliness alone.

Perhaps the intention of Nature, in permitting such vermin to annoy mankind, is to induce them to the practice of this virtue.

One common cause of putrid and malignant fevers is the want of cleanliness. These fevers commonly being among the inhabitants of close dirty houses, who breathe bad air, take little exercise, eat unwholesome food, and wear dirty clothes. There the infection is generally hatched, which spreads far and wide, to the destruction of many. Hence cleanliness may be considered as an object of public attention. It is not sufficient that I be clean myself, while the want of it in my neighbour affects my health as well as her own. If dirty people cannot be removed as a common nuisance, they ought at least to be avoided as infectious. All who regard their health should keep at a distance, even from their habitations. In places where great numbers of people are collected, cleanliness becomes of the utmost importance.

It is well known that infectious diseases are caused by tainted air. Everything, therefore, which tends to pollute the air, or spread the infection, ought with the utmost care to be avoided.

For this reason, in great towns, no filth of any kind should be permitted to lie upon the streets. We are sorry to say that the importance of general cleanliness in this respect does by no means seem to be sufficiently understood. It were well if the lower classes of the inhabitants of Great Britain would imitate their neighbours the Dutch in their assiduity in cleansing their streets, houses, &c.

Nothing can be more agreeable to the senses, or to the honour of the inhabitants or conducive to their health, than a clean town; nor does anything impress a stranger sooner with disrespectfulness of any people than its opposite. It is remarkable that, in most eastern countries, cleanliness make a great part of their religion. The Mahometan, as well as the Jewish religion, enjoins various bathings, washings and purifications. No doubt these were designed to represent inward purity; but they are at the same time calculated for the preservation of health.

However whimsical these washings may appear to some, few things would seem more to prevent diseases than a proper attention to many of them.

Were every person, for example, after handling a dead body, visiting the sick, etc., to wash before he went into company, or sat down to meat, he would run less hazard either of catching the infection himself, or communicating it to others.

Frequent washing not only removes the filth which adheres to the skin, but likewise promotes the perspiration, braces the body, and enlivens the spirits. Even washing the feet tends greatly to preserve health. The perspiration and dirt with which these parts are frequently covered, cannot fail to obstruct their pores. This piece of cleanliness would often prevent colds and fevers. Were people to bathe their feet and hands in warm water at night, after being exposed to cold or wet through the day, they would seldom experience any of the effects from these causes which often prove fatal.

In places where great numbers of sick people are kept, cleanliness ought most religiously to be observed. The very smell in such places is often sufficient to make one sick. It is easy to imagine what effect that is likely to have upon the diseased.

A person in health has a greater chance to become sick, than a sick person has to get well, in an hospital or infirmary where cleanliness is neglected. Even our own

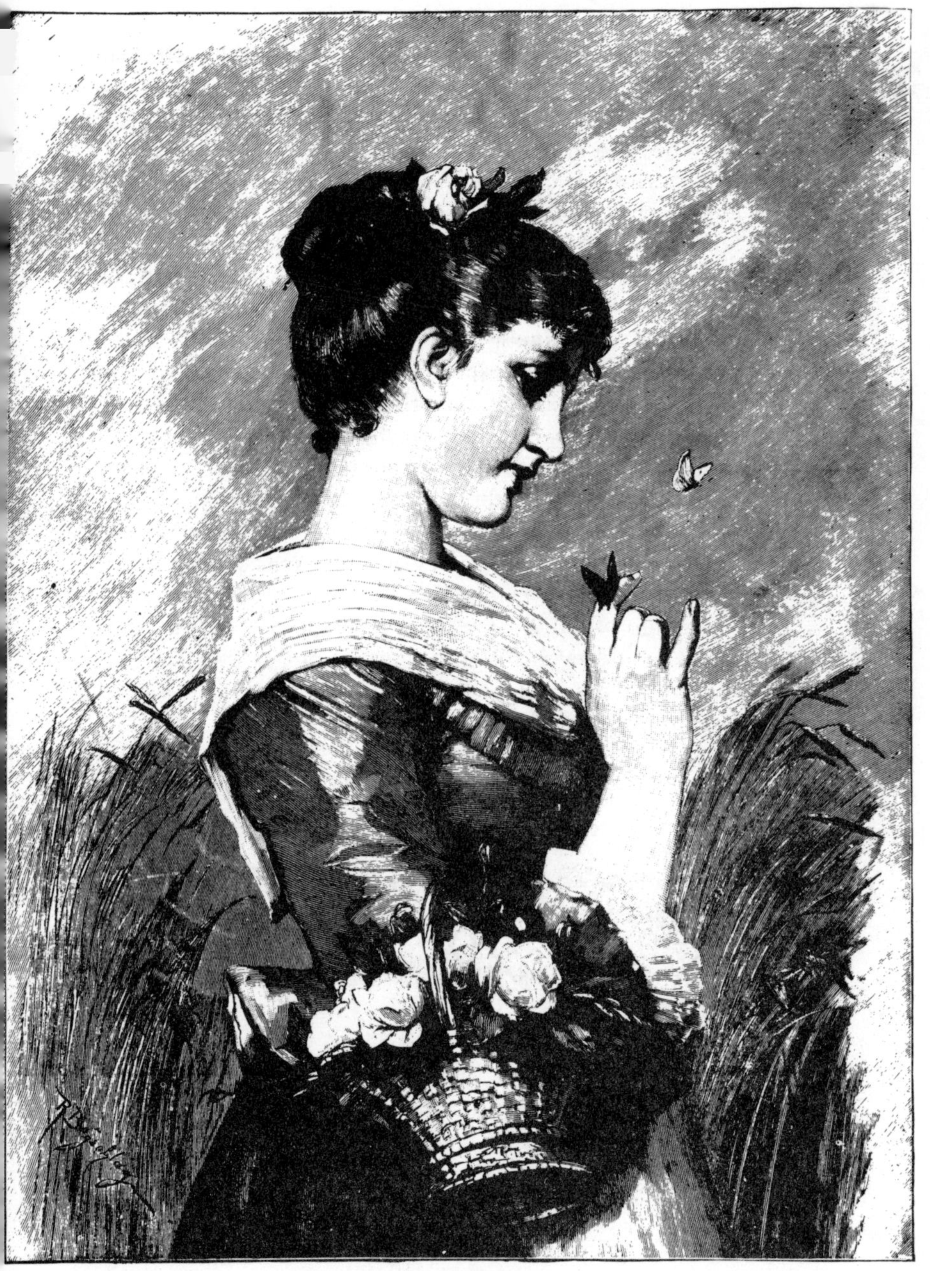

THE BUTTERFLY.

feelings are a sufficient proof of the necessity of cleanliness. How refreshed, how cheerful and agreeable does one feel on being washed and dressed, especially when these have been long neglected.

Superior cleanliness sooner attracts our regard than even finery itself, and often gains esteem where the other fails.

Influence of Cleanliness.—"I have more than once expressed my conviction that the humanizing influence of habits of cleanliness, and of those decent observations which imply self-respect—the best, indeed the only foundation of respect for others—has never been sufficiently acted on. A clean, fresh, and well-ordered house exercises over its inmates a moral no less than a physical influence, and has a direct tendency to make the members of a family, sober, peaceable, and considerate of the feelings and happiness of each other; nor is it difficult to trace a connection between habitual feelings of this sort and the formation of habits of respect for property, for the laws in general, and even for those higher duties and obligations the observance of which no laws can enforce."—Dr. Southwood Smith.

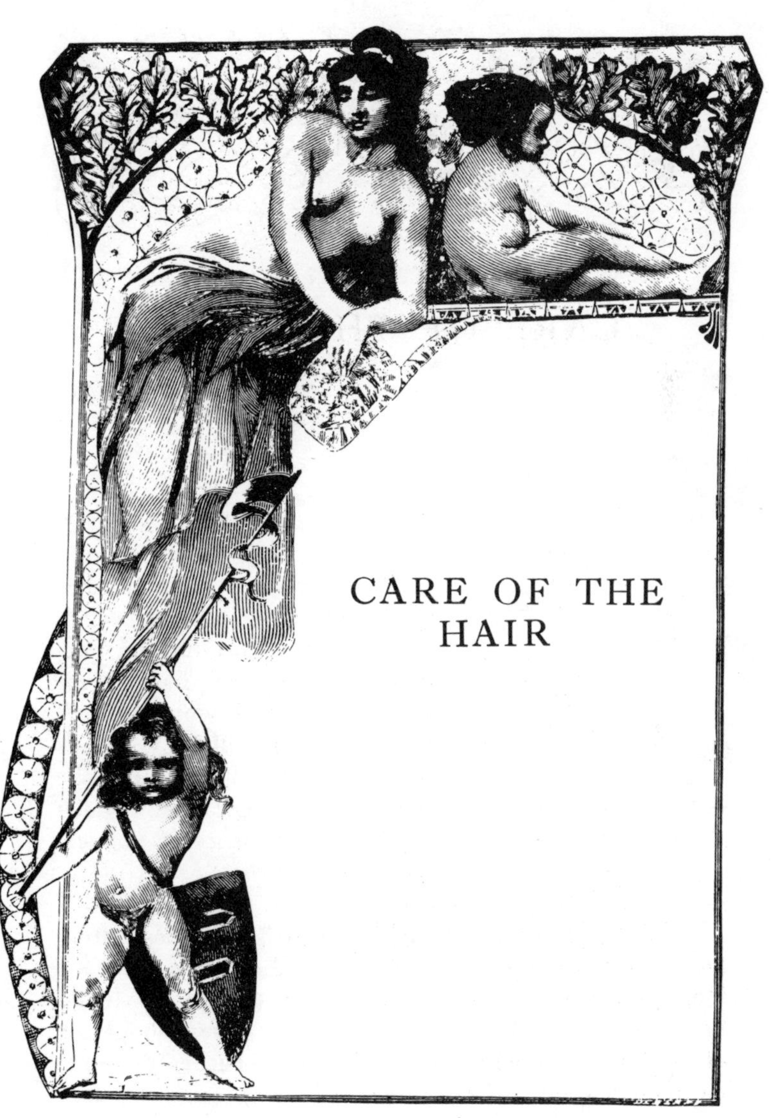

CARE OF THE
HAIR

CARE OF THE HAIR

No woman who values her appearance can afford to neglect her hair, for a fine, well-kept head of hair forms indeed a "woman's crowning glory," whereas dull-looking, ill-kept tresses tend to show more than anything else that she lacks that dainty and scrupulous care of her person which should prove one of the chief characteristics of her sex.

BRUSHING THE HAIR.

The hair should be thoroughly brushed for at least from five to eight minutes each morning and evening, and even longer if it is particularly thick and luxuriant. Care should be taken in the selection of the brushes. These should be of medium hardness—extremely hard brushes do more harm than good. A moderately stiff brush might be used for the hair, and a softer one for the scalp. Part the hair in two divisions from the centre of the forehead to the nape of the neck, then brush it at each side with firm, even, and rapid but not unduly hasty strokes. Few women understand the knack of hair-brushing, and more harm than good is done by an unduly harsh treatment with the brush. The brushing should be sufficiently brisk and vigorous to set the oil glands of the scalp in action. A healthy glow is felt over the head and scalp when the brushing is properly done.

COMBING THE HAIR.

It is as well to take out the tangles with the comb before brushing, taking care not to break the hair by pulling too hard. The teeth of the comb should not be too sharp; they should be firm and strong, however, and not easily breakable. Tortoise shell combs are the best, but these are not within the reach of every purse. Very good combs can be obtained for the expenditure of from 1s. 6d. to 2s.; but great care should be taken in their selection. The scalp should never be scraped with the comb, as this induces irritation and dandruff; neither should "back-combing," which is the name given to the process of fluffing out the hair by combing it back from the ends to the roots, in order to give the appearance of an added thickness, be much practised.

After thoroughly brushing and combing the hair at night it is best to do it up in one or two very loose plaits, in order to give it a much needed rest from the strain to which it has been subjected by the exigencies of the coiffure during the day-time. When the hair is tightly braided it cannot enjoy the benefit of this rest.

Much benefit can be derived from gently massaging the scalp with the tips of the fingers, using a quick, circular movement. Part the hair in the middle, massage gently from and round the parting, then separate the hair in strands, and massage the scalp from and round the smaller partings thus made. The friction so caused stimulates the oil glands, and does much to promote their healthy action. This massage may take place night or morning, but preferably in the morning, when the scalp is not tired. For very dry hair a little cocoa-butter might be applied with the tips of the fingers during the massaging process; it should be rubbed gently into the scalp and not allowed to go over the hair.

WASHING THE HAIR.

Too frequent washing of the hair is injurious, as it has the effect of removing the natural oil. No hard-and-fast rule can be laid down as to how often the hair should be washed; it is a matter which depends upon the nature and quantity of the hair and the condition of the scalp. People with abnormally greasy hair, for instance, require to wash it once a fortnight or three weeks to keep it in a good condition; whilst dwellers in the town are compelled to wash their hair more often than people who live in the country.

On the other hand, people with dry hair should wash it as seldom as is compatible with perfect cleanliness. A good plan for those whose hair tends to dryness is to rub oil well into the scalp twenty-four hours before washing. This will obviate any tendency of the hair to become harsh and brittle after the shampoo. One important point to remember is that soap should never be rubbed on to the hair during the washing process. The best way to

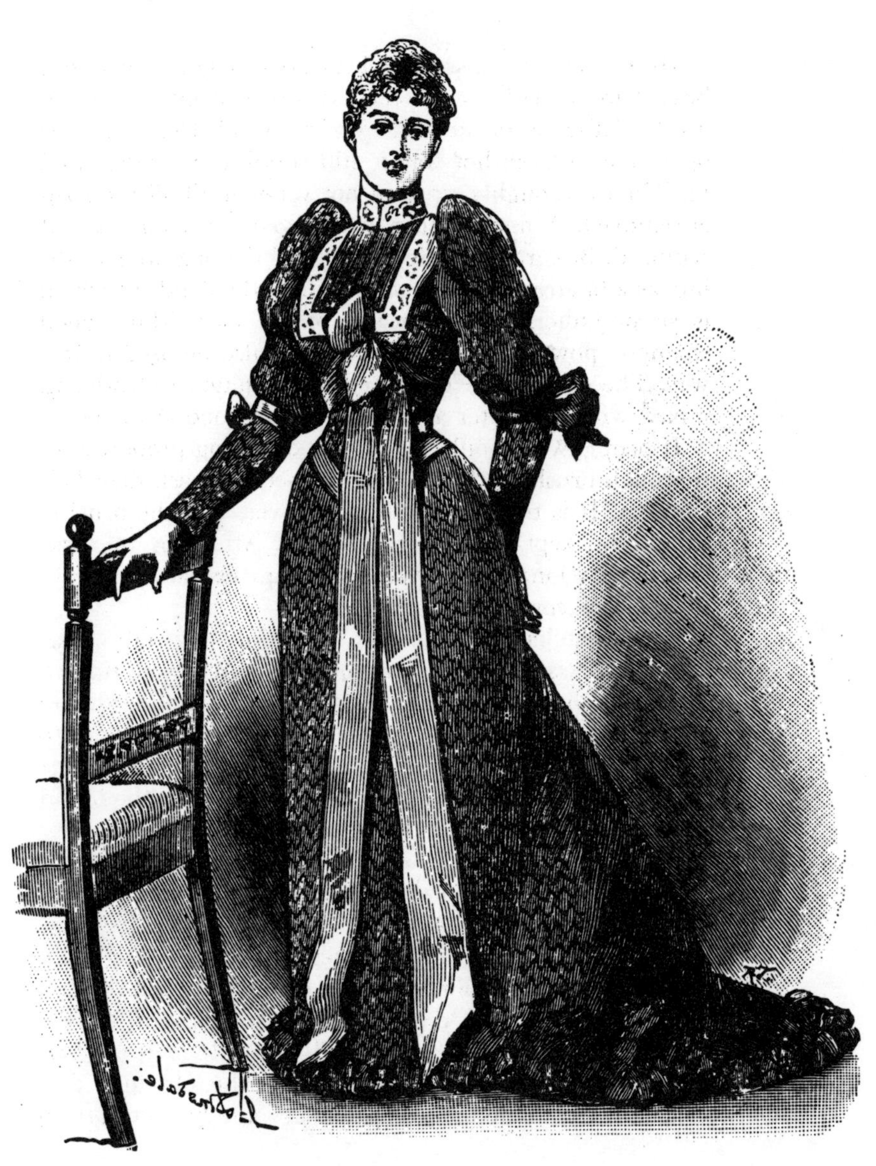

wash the hair is to dissolve a little good soap in hot water, beat it into a lather, and then rub it well into the scalp until a lather is formed all over the head. Continue this operation in fresh hot water, still rubbing the lather well in. Then thoroughly rinse in hot water until all the soap is removed. A final rinsing can be given in cold water if required. Be careful to thoroughly dry the hair after washing, as a failure to do this often causes the dandruff which is so prejudicial to the health of the hair. Many good shampoo powders are sold which can also be used in this way. The yolks of one or two eggs beaten up to a froth and mixed with hot water also make a very good shampoo.

If people would only realize the cleansing properties of thorough brushing they would not need to wash their hair so often. It is most important, however, that the brushes should be kept scrupulously clean. Attention to these details go a long way towards keeping the hair and scalp in a healthy condition.

Where the hair is inclined to be unduly dry and brittle, a little Macassar Oil or cocoa-butter should be well rubbed into the scalp twice a week. The former preparation should be used sparingly, two or three drops being sufficient to impart a delightful gloss. For unduly greasy hair a little bay rum rubbed into the roots twice a week will be found to have beneficial results in most cases.

Soda should never be used in washing the hair, for although it gives it a pretty, fluffy appearance, and tends to make fair hair look fairer, yet it is very injurious, having a most drying and irritating effect upon the scalp, causing the hair to split and break, and after a time to fall, if constantly used. Occasional tipping (i.e. cutting the ends of the hair) and singeing is beneficial when the hair is broken and the ends uneven, but the old idea that constant tipping and singeing was absolutely necessary to

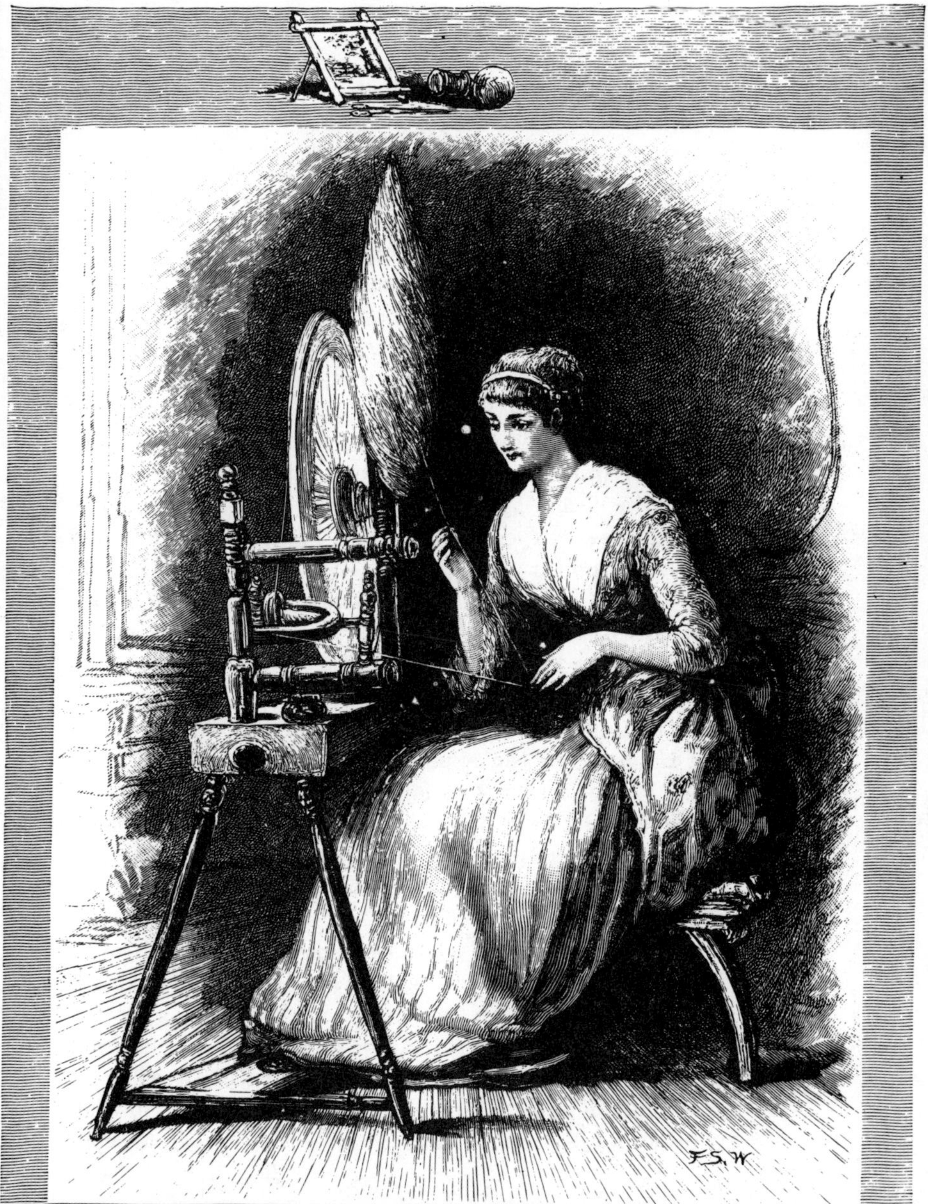

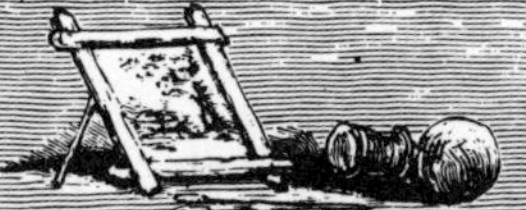

Industry.

keep the hair in good condition is now altogether exploded.

TOILET BRUSHES.

It is very important to keep hair brushes very clean. They should always be kept under cover and not allowed to lie about exposed to the dust. Then wash them once a week or as often as occasion requires. Put sufficient hot water into a bowl or basin to cover the bristles of the brush and add a good teaspoonful of borax, a lump of soda, or enough ammonia to make the water smell rather strongly. Allow this to become luke-warm. Remove all hairs from the brush and dab it up and down in the water until it looks quite clean. The water must not be allowed to come over the back of the brush, or it is liable to loosen it and destroy the polish on the wood. Rinse thoroughly in cold water, which will prevent the bristles from becoming soft. Shake out the water, wipe the back of the brush with a towel, and dry as quickly as possible in the open air or in a warm atmosphere.

Soda should not be used for fine and expensive brushes as it might spoil the appearance of the backs; borax or ammonia are safer materials.

Polished wood or ebony backs can be rubbed up with a little furniture polish when the brushes are dry; tortoiseshell or ivory backs with a little sweet oil.

TO WASH COMBS.

Make a lather of soap and water. Take a small nail brush with crisp but not unduly hard bristles, and apply the soapsuds to the comb, brushing from the back of the comb to the edges of the teeth (left to right) with a brisk even movement. This brings out the dirt more effectively than by brushing the comb lengthways. Rinse well in cold

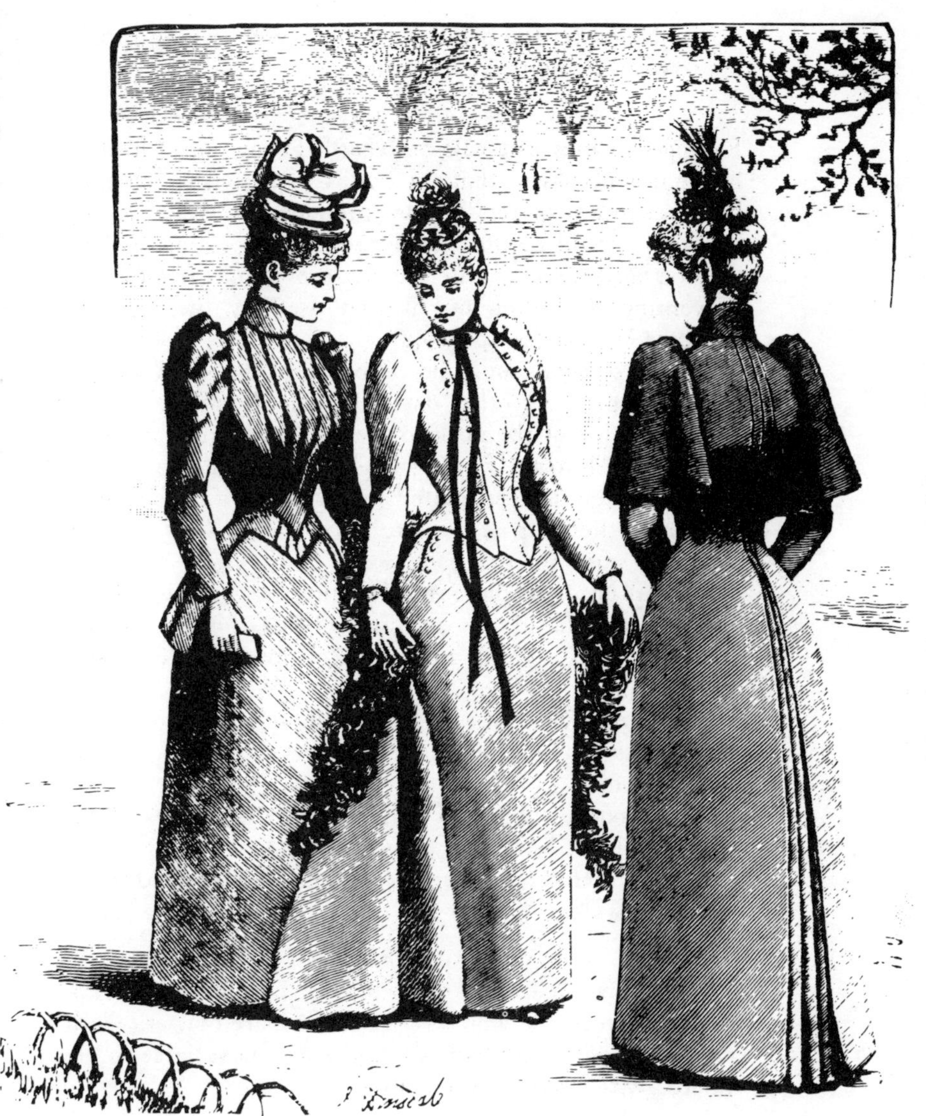

water. Never let the comb lie in hot water—doing this is apt to bend it and make it brittle.

FALLING HAIR.

Falling hair may as a rule be regarded a sign of ill health, hence it is necessary that any bodily condition which may be discovered as tending to produce the affliction in question should be duly corrected. Among lotions which may be used for strenghtening the growth of the hair and preventing its falling out is that used by the late Sir Erasmus Wilson (see page 92).

A little of this should be rubbed into the scalp with a small sponge every other day. The hair should be parted from the nape of the neck to the forehead, and the tonic well rubbed into the parting thus made. Then the hair at the sides should be separated into strands, and the tonic applied to the scalp at the smaller partings. This tonic is especially good for dry hair.

For greasy hair the following preparation should be used. Of Cantharides 2 drachms; of Oil of Lemon $\frac{1}{2}$ an ounce; of Red Lavender 2 drachms; of Spirits of Rosemary up to 4 ounces.

A little paraffin well rubbed into the scalp at night-time with the tips of the fingers in some cases acts as a very efficient tonic.

One important point to remember is that the hair and scalp should be well shampooed before first beginning to use a hair tonic if the utmost benefit is to be derived from its use.

GREY HAIRS.

As a rule fair-haired women do not become grey with advancing years as soon as their dark-haired sisters, and the woman with dark hair is also the one most liable to be afflicted with premature greyness.

Premature greyness can in many cases be arrested, whilst the greyness that comes of advancing years must necessarily take its course. The woman whose locks show a tendency to become grey before she has attained the age of thirty should at once consult a good hair specialist, and so try to nip the mischief in the bud.

Grey hair, like wrinkles, are often caused by constant worry or disorder of the nervous system, and the general health requires attention if the progress of the wintry locks is to be arrested. It has been said that constantly washing the hair with soda is very conducive to premature greyness. An excessively dry condition of the scalp should be avoided, and some good nourishing hair tonic regularly applied.

FALSE HAIR.

False hair enters so largely into the scheme of fashionable hair-dressing that a few words on the subject will not be amiss. False curls, plaits, twists of all kinds are requisitioned in the present-day coiffures, even by those whose locks are naturally abundant. The wearing of masses of false curls over the natural hair cannot but be harmful to the scalp, which becomes unduly heated as the fresh air, so essential to the health of the hair, is excluded. The weight of a light, false plait or twist wound round the head is almost imperceptible, and so additions of this kind to the natural locks cannot do much harm, but it is heavy masses of curls and coils which should be avoided. If some addition is required to the tresses, the best way is to save up one's hair combings until there are sufficient for a plait, or switch or coil, and send them to a good hair-dresser to be made up. The combings must be kept in a well-closed box, and they should not be kept too long before being made up, or they will become dull and lose their colour.

Whatever care may be given to other details of the toilette will be nullified to a certain extent by an ill-dressed head of hair. The clever woman realizes that her looks depend a great deal upon suitable arrangement of her tresses, and she takes pains to dress her hair to suit her face. When she possesses a pretty forehead and well-arched eyebrows she dresses her hair well away from the brows, knowing that it is the style which will suit her best.

If her face is unduly long, with prominent features, she shuns the middle parting, which could only add to its length. If, on the other hand, it inclines to undue square-ness or plumpness, she avoids the pompadour, which would only tend to accentuate these defects.

There is nothing more unsightly than ill-kempt, straggly tresses, unless it is the hair brushed stiffly and strained so tightly as to give an appearance of being pulled out by the roots.

Those who are wise realize that the hair is a frame, as it were, to the face, which can be made to beautify the picture it surrounds, or else to detract very materially from its beauty.

The best coiffures invariably convey an idea of natural-ness of arrangement, although artificial waving and other expedients may have been resorted to in order to bring about the desired results.

WAVING AND CURLING THE HAIR.

It is not given to us all to have naturally wavy or curly hair. For those who are so fortunate as to possess it, the difficulties of hair-dressing are materially lessened, for wavy hair has a way of arranging itself naturally and becomingly with very little care. It has the advantage also of never looking really untidy, although "artistic untidiness" is generally the effect of curly tresses, for the little curls rebel at being unduly restricted by hairpins and ribbons, and have a knack of breaking away from the restraint of these accessories of the coiffure upon the least provocation, but with the happiest results.

Where the hair is inclined to be fluffy much may be done to simulate the natural wave. Of all forms of artificial waving that of doing up the hair in good waving pins is perhaps the most satisfactory for the woman who dresses her own hair.

Nowadays, it is true, very excellent waving and curling tongs and irons are sold, but to use them satisfactorily requires the knack of a trained coiffeur. The home use of curling and waving irons of all kinds should be discouraged, for the hair is often invariably impoverished by constant burning with hot tongs. It requires an expert to use them properly. If you must use them, take a course of lessons in waving from a good hairdresser, or, better still, go to the hairdresser once a week or once a fortnight to have the hair waved. A wave will last a week or even a fortnight with fluffy hair, and the hairdresser's charge as a rules does not come to more than 1s. 6d.

THE USE OF WAVING AND CURLING PINS.

Of curling and waving pins those sold by Messrs. Hinde are perhaps amongst the best. They can be obtained from almost any hairdresser or draper in the United Kingdom, and are very easy to use. Upon getting up in the morning separate the part of the hair which is to be waved into strands, and twist each strand round a waver. By the time the toilet is complete and it is time to begin the coiffure, upon taking out the pins it will be found that the hair is well and naturally waved. If the hair is inclined to be abnormally greasy, it will not wave quite so quickly, then it will be necessary sometimes to leave the pins in over-night. This should not be done often, however, as the hair needs rest during the night-time, and should not be sub-jected to any unnecessary strain if this can be avoided. A little rum or spirit of any kind rubbed on to the hair before waving will very often act as a most effective curl-ing fluid; often also by slightly warming the pins in the flame of a candle or a gas jet before using, the hair will be found to wave much more quickly. Fringes are very little worn at the present day; a few stray curls here and there on the forehead are the utmost concession made by fashion to those who find a fringe of some kind necessary. One of Hinde's curlers will be all that is necessary for the curling of the present-day fringes. Where the hair is unusually dank and greasy two might be used, but care must be taken to avoid the very stiffly curled fringe which is now terribly demode.

DRESSING THE HAIR.

In almost every successful coiffure the front and back portions of the hair are dressed separately. After having waved the hair, part it first of all from ear to ear. This will separate the front and back portions.

Comb up the back portion towards the centre of the back of the head, and if the hair is long tie it in the required position, or fasten it with a hair-binder. It is better not to tie short hair, as more can be made of it if left loose. Then take the front portion, shaking it down over the face, and comb it well. If the pompadour effect is required, separate the hair into three divisions, gently fluff the centre part of the division with the comb, turn it up and fasten into position with an ornamental comb. Do the same with each of the side pieces, taking care not to leave a parting on either side. With fluffy hair the pompa-

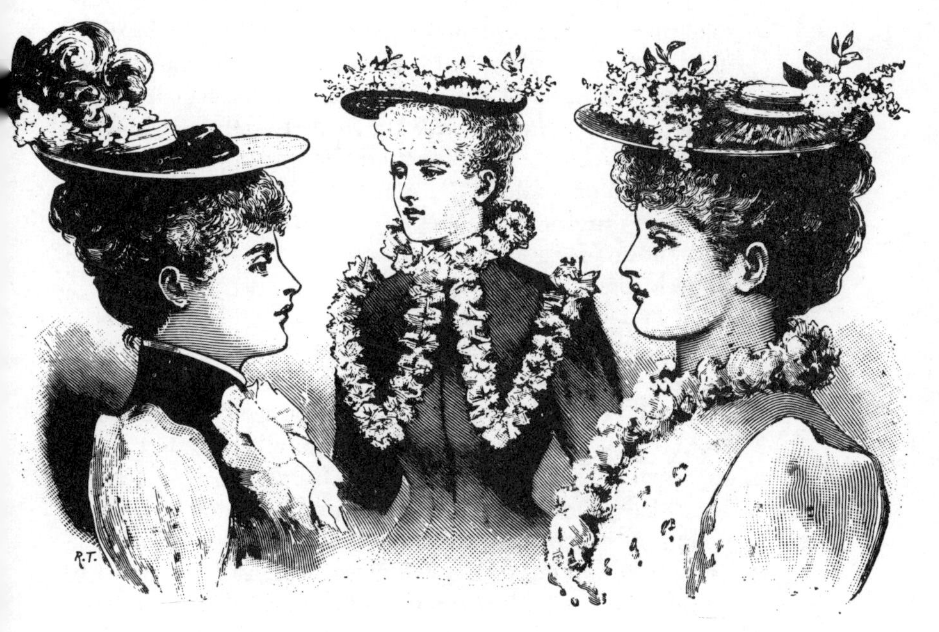

dour effect can be achieved without the aid of a pad; with very straight hair a light pad is necessary—it must be a very light one and the hair must not be strained too tightly over it.

If a parting is required, part it in two in the middle, take up each side separately, gently push the hair forward, and keep it in place with side-combs. The harsh, even parting is a thing of the past nowadays; the hair is always parted loosely, and a little wave made to fall over the forehead on each side. If preferred the parting can be made to come to one side.

These preliminary steps carefully attended to, the foundation of a good coiffure is made; the hair can now be done in the style preferred.

FASHIONABLE COIFFURES.

During the last winter season, a style of hairdressing known as the "Turban Coiffure" was introduced into England from Paris, and became pretty generally adopted by all those who wished to be "in the fashion." This style of head-dress, however, though admirably suited to our fair neighbours across the Channel, was by no means universally becoming to English faces. The foundation of the coiffure was a large turban frame which fitted the head like a cap; the hair was drawn through a hole at the base of the frame and arranged over it in a flat chignon or turban, whilst a straight band of hair drawn round the chignon so formed completed the coiffure. By reason of its general unbecomingness to English faces the reign of the "Turban" was shortlived. English hairdressers met together in conference to deliberate whether it was not possible to design coiffures in England instead of adopting the Paris styles. As a result of their deliberations, a typical English coiffure has been introduced which bids fair to lead the fashion for some time to come.

The curls which were so great a feature of the fashion in coiffures a few years ago have been revived, only with a difference. They are much larger, and are generally built on frames still retaining something of the turban shape. These are encircled by a coil of hair drawn in many cases through tortoiseshell rings, which form part of the back-comb. As an alternative a straight flat slide is worn at the base of the hair. For evening dress three short ringlets are allowed to fall over the nape of the neck at the back. These ringlets are as a rule absent from the coiffure in the day-time, although for very dressy occasions they may sometimes be worn; on these occasions, however, the dress collar would have to be low.

The arrangement of the very dressy form of the new coiffure can seldom be effected by a woman herself without the help of a lady's-maid, and some extraneous aid to her own locks in the form of curls, switches, &c. The simpler forms, however, do not require so much elaboration, although the same idea is maintained, and a woman can effect the fashionable arrangement of her tresses without even the aid of a hairframe in the following way.

If the hair is long and plentiful, after arranging and waving the front portion, take up all the hair at the centre of the head at the back and tie it or fasten it with one of Hinde's hairbinders in the centre of the head, leaving the under portion of the hair hanging loose over the shoulders. Then separate the bound portion into strands, making several large curls, take up the under-portion and coil it loosely round the curls, fix one of the fashionable hair-slides in the hair just above the nape of the neck, and the coiffure is complete.

With short hair, the hair should not be bound. It should be separated into two portions in the way already described; the under-portion should be well pinned back while the upper portion is being curled, then it should be divided into two strands, which should be made to cross one over the other at the back and twisted round on either side of the head to give the appearance of one complete strand.

A woman sometimes finds it very difficult to make the fashionable curls by twisting strands of hair over her fingers; the curls are apt to break and become loose when made in this manner. Messrs. Burnet & Temple Ltd., have brought out a very simple and ingenious device by which curls and puffs can be made with the least amount of trouble. This consists of a small wooden stick round which the hair is rolled; the stick is fitted with grooves through which a safety hairpin is inserted, fastening the curl in place when the stick is removed.

It must be remembered that fashions in millinery have a most decided influence upon fashions in hairdressing; a woman must nowadays dress her hair to suit her hat, and the latest evolution of the coiffure may be ascribed to the vogue for very large and picturesque head-gear which has prevailed for so long. As a relief from large hats, the turban toques are equally fashionable, and the simpler form of hairdressing described is suitable for either the one form of millinery or the other, the only difference being that the bouffant and waved effects at the sides should be more elaborate when wearing a large hat than with the toque. In this latter case the side dressing may be comparatively simple.

COMBS AND SLIDES.

Ornamental combs and slides play an important part in the present styles of hairdressing. The slide is particularly useful as well as an ornamental accessory. Placed as it is at the back of the coiffure, it prevents the hair becoming caught in the hooks or buttons of a high collar, and helps to keep the curls trim and tidy. Combs have very deep, wide borders, which serve to convey the appearance of hair-slides when placed in the hair. Very large tortoise-shell hairpins are also worn; in fact, it may be said that as waving and curling is a feature of present-day hair-dressing, the popularity of combs, fancy pins, and other similar accessories will largely increase, as they are most effective in accentuating the deep waves and curls, and at the same time serve to keep them in place, imparting a "finished" appearance to the coiffure.

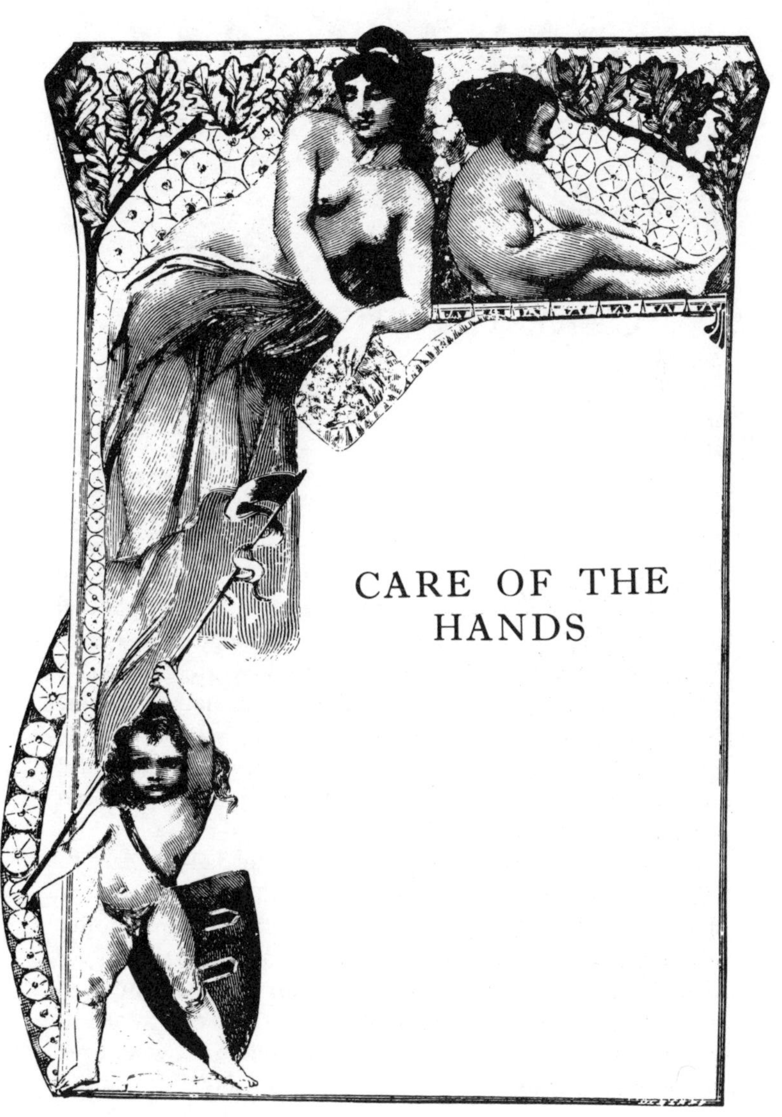

CARE OF THE HANDS

CARE OF THE HANDS

ANY A woman who is on the whole particular in regard to her general appearance is apt to neglect the care of her hands. This is a great mistake, as ill-kept hands and nails are unsightly in the extreme, whilst a well-groomed hand is not only pleasant to the eye, but is also one of the best indications of refinement a woman can possess.

Housework is often made the excuse for lack of care in this direction. The average woman is apt to entertain the idea that well-kept hands are incompatible with the proper fulfilment of domestic duties. This is quite a fallacy, for with a little care the busy housewife can keep her hands in as good condition as the lady of leisure, who can afford to spend half-an-hour or an hour at her manicurist whenever she feels so inclined.

Thin rubber surgeon's gloves should be worn when doing work which necessitates the hands being constantly in and out of the water, such as washing dishes, scrubbing, &c. A pair of old gloves should always be kept in readiness for wear when dusting, sweeping, or performing other similar duties. They should, if possible, be a size too large, so as not to restrain the circulation in any way. Gloves should also be worn when engaged in gardening and other out-of-door work.

Cleanliness is, of course, the first essential in this portion of the toilet. The hands should be well washed in good soap and warm water softened with a little borax or some good toilet vinegar night and morning, and, whenever necessary, during the day. A good nail-brush with firm bristles should be used for scrubbing the nails, and pumice stone or lemon or both for removing the stains from the hands and fingers. When the hands become soiled and greasy after the performance of household duties, a little cold cream or white vaseline should be rubbed well into them before and after washing, in order to keep the skin smooth and soft. On home washing days, when there is a great deal of laundry work to be done, after being immersed for a long time in the wash-tub the hands are apt to assume a rather harsh, wrinkled appearance. This can be cured by dipping them into a little vinegar; they should then be rubbed with cold cream, as after the performance of other household duties.

After washing and drying the hands before going to bed at night, glycerine and rose-water, or red lavender, mixed in the proportions of two parts glycerine to one of red lavender, should be rubbed into the skin. To do this thoroughly it is well to rub the mixture well into the palms and then rub the hands together as in washing.

When the work of the house has been abnormally heavy, and, in spite of all precautions, the hands have become a little rough, it is advisable to wear a pair of large chamois leather gloves at night, or a pair of old kid gloves one or two sizes too large. Gloves of the normal size would not do. They would restrict the healthy circulation of the blood, and red, not white hands would be the result.

DRYING THE HANDS.

The importance of thoroughly drying the hands after washing cannot be too highly estimated. A neglect of this causes the skin to become red and coarsened, and in winter time chapped hands and often chilblains are the result. Many a busy housewife is content, after hurriedly washing her hands, to dry them perhaps on a kitchen roller towel, the latter being most probably wet already through constant use. Every bit as much care should be taken in drying the hands as in washing them. They should be dried first with a ordinary linen towel, and then well rubbed with a soft Turkish towel. An added precaution to take would be to dust them over with fine oatmeal, a little Fuller's earth or any good toilet powder.

CARE OF THE NAILS, MANICURE.

Every woman should be able to manicure her hands and nails for herself. The process is a very simple one and only requires a little care and the proper implements.

The following articles are necessary for the use of the home manicurist:—
A packet of orange sticks for pushing back the skin.
A small nail file.
A small brush.
A pair of curved nail scissors.

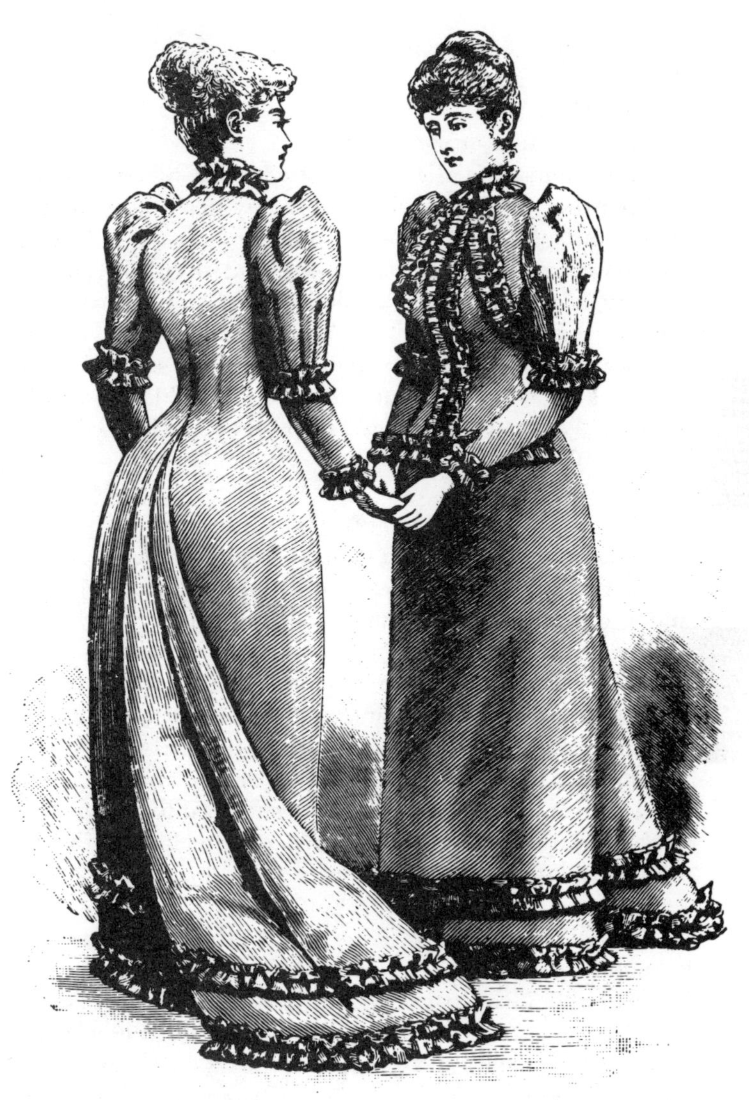

Some good cold cream.
A box of nail powder.
A nail polisher.
Some fine emery or sand-paper.

Cases containing the orange sticks, nail file and brush and polisher can be obtained from any perfumers for the small sum of 10½d. or one shilling, whilst most leather merchants sell compact little cases containing the curved scissors as well for from 2s. 6d. to 3s. 6d. The manicure powder can be obtained from all perfumers and chemists in boxes of from sixpence upwards. It is as well of course to get as good a set of implements as possible, as a little additional money spent on the original outlay will pay in the long run.

TO MANICURE THE NAILS.

Take some warm water and make a good lather of soap-suds. Add a few drops of eau-de-Cologne or toilet vinegar and the juice of half a lemon. Soak the fingers for from five to ten minutes in the soap-suds. This process has the effect of softening the nails so that they are ready for attention. Then after having rubbed a little cold cream well into the skin round the base of the nails. By doing this those half-moons which are so dainty and attractive a feature of well-kept nails are brought into view. The cuticle of the nail should never be touched with the scissors unless it is absolutely necessary to use them to cut a hang-nail.

The nails should now be cut round the edges if necessary and filed into shape with the little file. The curve of the nail should be trimmed to follow that of the finger-tips. The ideal nail is of an oval form, and although we do not all have the good fortune to possess oval finger-tips, a little careful manipulation in the trimming of the nails will do a great deal in giving them an oval appearance as far as possible. Constant practice works wonders in the proper manipulation of the nail file.

After the nails have been carefully filed, a little of the sand-paper should be used to smooth away the rough edges.

Finally, the nail powder should be applied with the brush, and the nails should be gently polished with the polisher. The latter consists of a little instrument somewhat in the shape of a miniature iron with the flat part covered with chamois leather. If no polisher is available, it is often sufficient to rub the nails against the palm of the hand.

After this treatment has been gone through, the nails will assume that pink and polished appearance which adds so much to their beauty, and which is quite easily attainable by the expenditure of a little care.

The manicuring process should be gone through at least once a week. Every day, however, the cuticle of the nail should be pushed back with the orange stick after washing, or even with the towel. The polisher should then be used with light rapid friction, and this daily attention will keep the nails in proper condition.

A very good substitute for ordinary nail polishing powder can be obtained from Messrs. Pritchard & Constance, of Haymarket, London. It is sold under the trademark of "Amami" Polishing Stone, for the moderate price of sixpence. "Amami" Nail-Polishing Stone is no trouble: merely rub on the moistened palm of the hand, first the stone, and then the finger nails; the thumb nails should be done separately. A lasting pearly polish appears at once. The substance of the stone, in addition to being quite harmless, tends to preserve in good condition both the nails and the cuticle.

Where the nails are unduly dry and brittle, a little olive

oil rubbed into them at night will do wonders in restoring
them to good condition.

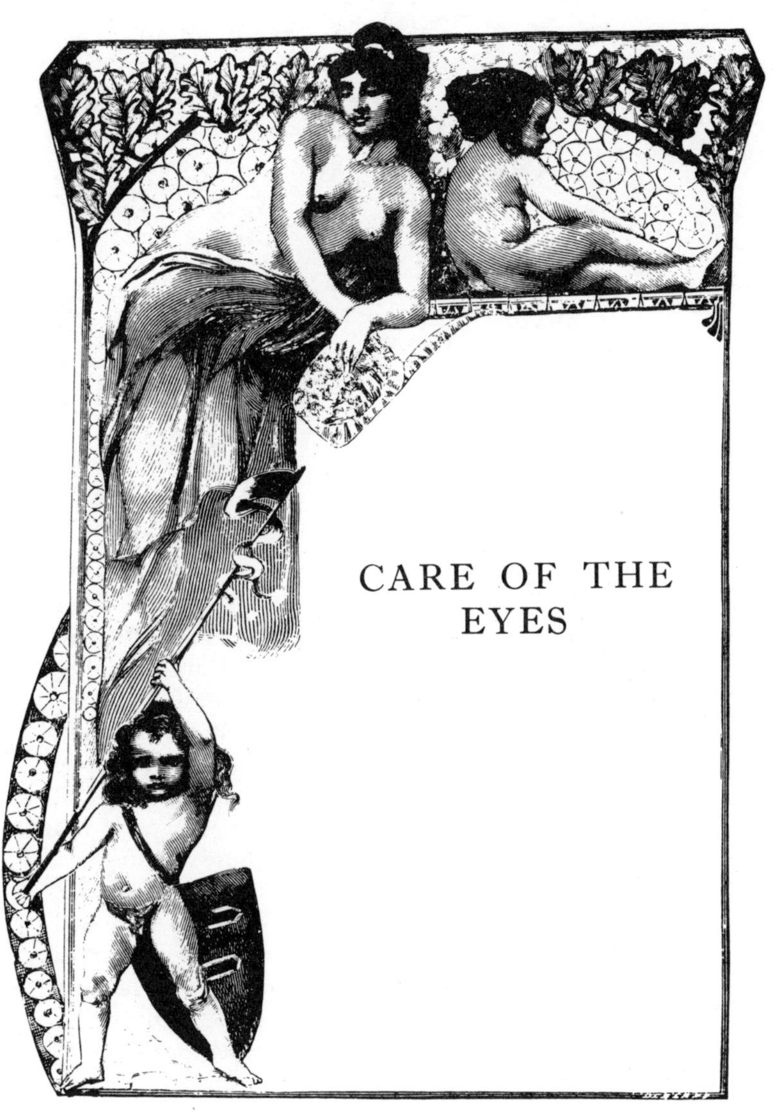

CARE OF THE EYES

CARE OF THE EYES

OT ONLY are the eyes the all-essential organs of sight, but they have also been described as the "Mirror of the Soul." They reflect our thoughts, our intellect, our emotions, and our sympathies, giving to the face that spiritualness which forms its chief beauty. They can be made indeed the most formidable weapon in the armoury of woman's charm, and yet they are the very organs of her body which she is the most inclined to abuse and neglect.

The average woman thinks nothing of straining her eyes over books or needlework in an indifferent light. It is bad for the eyes even in a good light to strain them over small print or minute stitches for hours at a stretch. The eyes require rest as much as the other organs of the body, and if they are required to do more than their fair share of work they are bound to suffer in the long run.

In the evening, when artificial light is required, be careful to sit with your back to the light, so that it is thrown on the pages of the book, and not straight into the eyeballs. The light should be shaded. Dark green shades are the most restful to the sight, and lamps and lights should be covered with them wherever possible.

From the point of view of our personal hygience the care of the eyes and eyebrows, eyelids and eyelashes, should receive daily consideration.

The eyes are naturally at their best, of course, when the health is at its best. Nothing can impart to the pupils the brilliancy of good health. Very often drugs such as belladonna are resorted to to give them the sparkle and shine which for some cause they lack. This is a most injurious practice, and can be productive of nothing but harm.

When washing in the morning care should be taken that the secretions which have accumulated in the corner of the eyes during sleep are removed. These, be it noted, should be washed out with warm water. It is inadvisable to rub into the corner of the eyes with a towel in order to dislodge the secretions, as inflammation is very often caused in this way. At night-time also care should be taken that the eyes are given their proper share of consideration in the evening toilet.

USE OF THE EYE-CUP.

When the secretions which accumulate round the eyes during the night are found to be so unduly heavy as to be difficult to dislodge in the morning, to thoroughly purify the eye it will be found necessary to have an eye-cup. This is a little glass cup made in the shape of the eyeball. It should be filled with warm water in which a pinch of boracic powder has been dissolved. Hold the cup towards the eye, lower the head slightly to meet it, and it will be found that the eye-cup fits round the eye exactly. Tilt the head backwards and forwards, holding the cup into position, and open and close the eyelid in the water until the eye is thoroughly cleansed. Dab gently with a small piece of soft rag to dry, and repeat the same treatment with the other eye. The eye-cup can also be used at night to remove the dust and dirt which have accumulated during the day. In all cases where the nature of the daily occupation forces the eyes to go through a heavy strain the daily use of the eye-cup will prove a most beneficial tonic.

When the eyes have been so severely strained that they are red and inflamed round the rims, and the secretions are so extensive that it is sometimes difficult to open the lids in the morning, a lotion should be used after bathing. This should be prescribed by a good oculist. In all cases of persistent trouble with the eyes an oculist should be at once consulted. There are people who, upon the first signs of eye-strain, rush to the nearest optician, buy a pair of glasses, and think that they have done all that is required. This mode of procedure may answer with luck, but most often it results in permanent injury to the eyesight. There is nothing more injurious for the eyes than unsuitable glasses. Glasses should only be made to the prescription of a good oculist who, after thorough examination and testing of the patient's sight, knows exactly what is required. Very often glasses are not required, and a simple lotion will set the trouble right. So those who, upon the first little trouble with their eyes, are inclined to at once buy spectacles, should be wise and find out first if they are really needed before they ruin their sight for life.

EYEBROWS AND EYELASHES.

Well-marked eyebrows and good lashes are invaluable

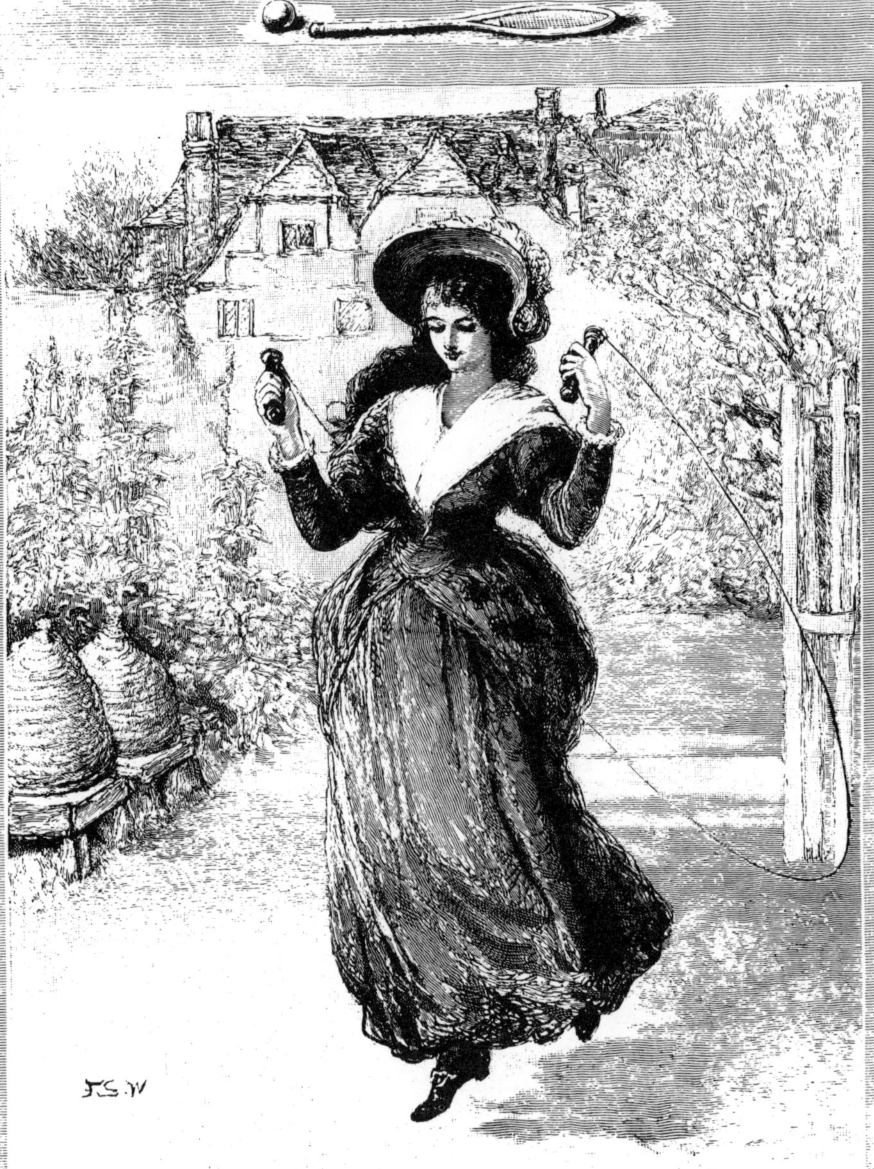

Recreation.

aids to beauty, and although it is not possible for us all to attain the high arched brows and long curling lashes which form the ideal of the artist, yet with care we can train our brows and lashes to something very near it.

Where the brows and lashes are thin, vaseline or cocoa-butter well rubbed into them at night serve to promote their growth; but the treatment must be persisted in regularly to produce results.

When the eyebrows are unduly straight, by careful manipulation with the fingers when applying the vaseline, and pinching the hair with a semi-circular movement upwards, they can be trained into something like the arched brows we all covet. The vaseline should be applied to the eyelashes gently and carefully, either with the tip of the first finger or the end of a match covered with a piece of soft rag. It should be applied under the lashes, which should be gently coaxed outwards and upwards to induce them to curl at the tips. When this has been done, dab the eyelids gently with a piece of clean soft rag to remove all superfluous vaseline, which, if allowed to remain, might cause the lashes to stick together.

The hair should never be dressed to fall very low over the forehead so as to cover the brows. A coiffure of this kind tends to wear away the eyebrows and impede their growth.

Brushing the brows with a small brow-brush night and morning goes a long way towards improving their appearance.

There is not much use in having pretty brows, however, if we mar them by continual frowning. The frowning habit grows upon one imperceptibly, and it is a habit very hard to correct. Persistent frowning brings those unsightly little lines between the brows which does so much to spoil their beauty. They can be removed in time with persistent care and treatment, but a habit once contracted is hard to get rid of, and no matter how often the little lines are effaced, if the frowning habit continues they will reappear.

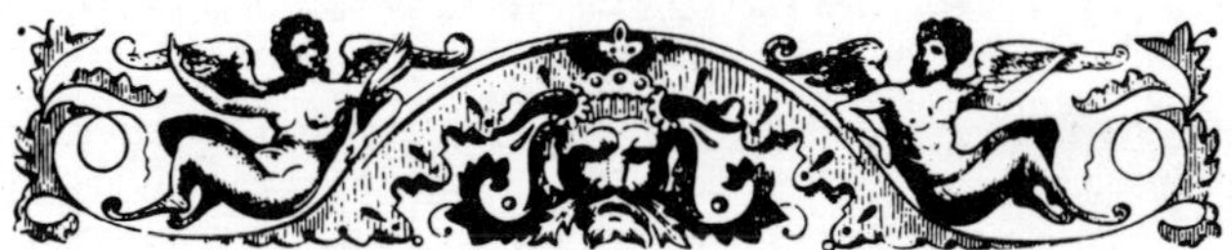

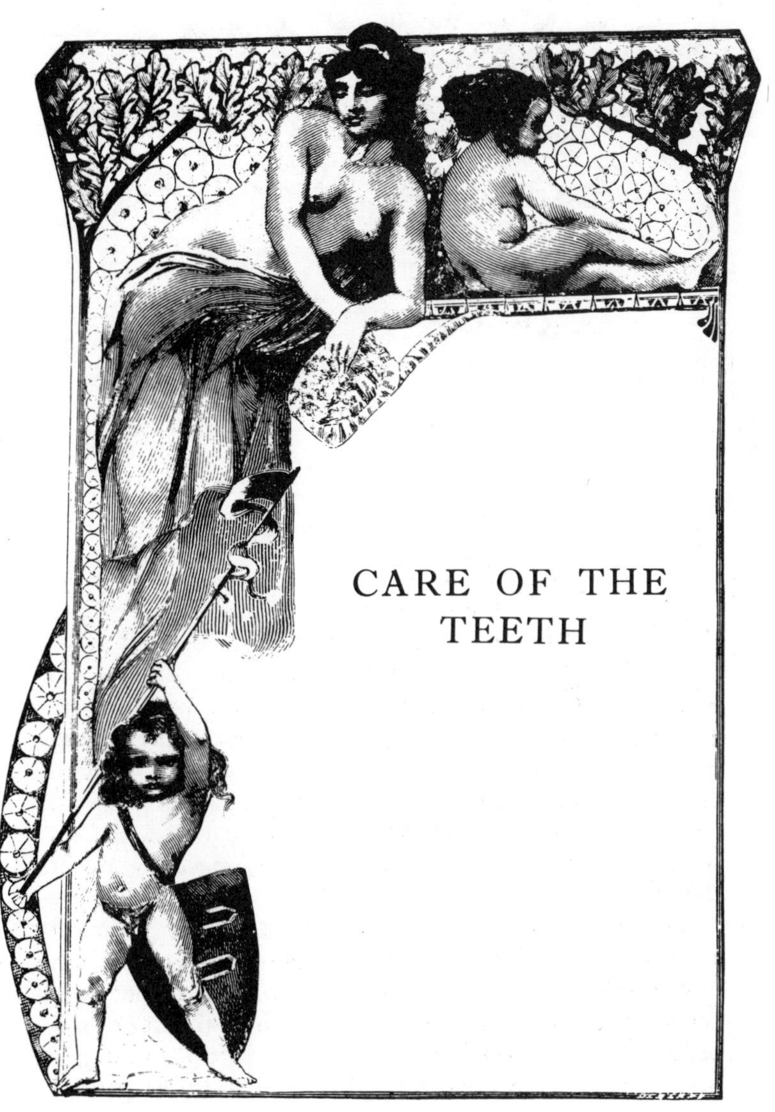

CARE OF THE
TEETH

CARE OF THE TEETH

TOO MUCH stress cannot be laid upon the extreme importance of the proper care of the teeth. Indigestion and other gastric troubles are often traced to decayed and defective teeth. To masticate food properly good teeth are of paramount importance. To keep the teeth and mouth clean is one of the surest methods of keeping them sound. Care should be taken, therefore, that all particles of food which collect between the teeth are dislodged by aid of the tooth-brush.

The teeth should be brushed at least twice a day, night and morning, and also after meals if possible. A good tooth powder should be used, and the teeth brushed not only across, but also up and down, the teeth of the upper jaw being brushed downwards, and those of the lower jaw being brushed upwards. Attention should also be paid to the gums. They should be brushed as carefully as the teeth. The mouth might be also rinsed with a good antiseptic mouth wash every evening. Calvert's Carbolic Tooth Powder or precipitated chalk are very good for cleansing purposes, and used in conjunction with a mouth wash, in accordance with the directions given, will serve to keep the mouth and teeth in a clean and wholesome condition. Where tartar accumulates upon the teeth to any great extent, it should be scraped off by a dentist. It is superfluous to add that when tooth decay does make its appearance the dentist should at once be consulted and the ill thoroughly remedied. It is not generally known that a milk diet is very injurious to the teeth, becoming acid on the gums, destroys the enamel. This may be obviated by using a good pinch of carbonate of soda in the water with which the teeth are brushed.

The care of her teeth is apt to be too much neglected by the average woman; and yet it is quite a simple matter to keep them clean and healthy, and a little care in this direction brings its reward an hundred-fold. Leaving all questions of health apart, bad and badly kept teeth spoil the prettiest face, whilst good, well-kept teeth have often the effect of redeeming a countenance from actual plainness.

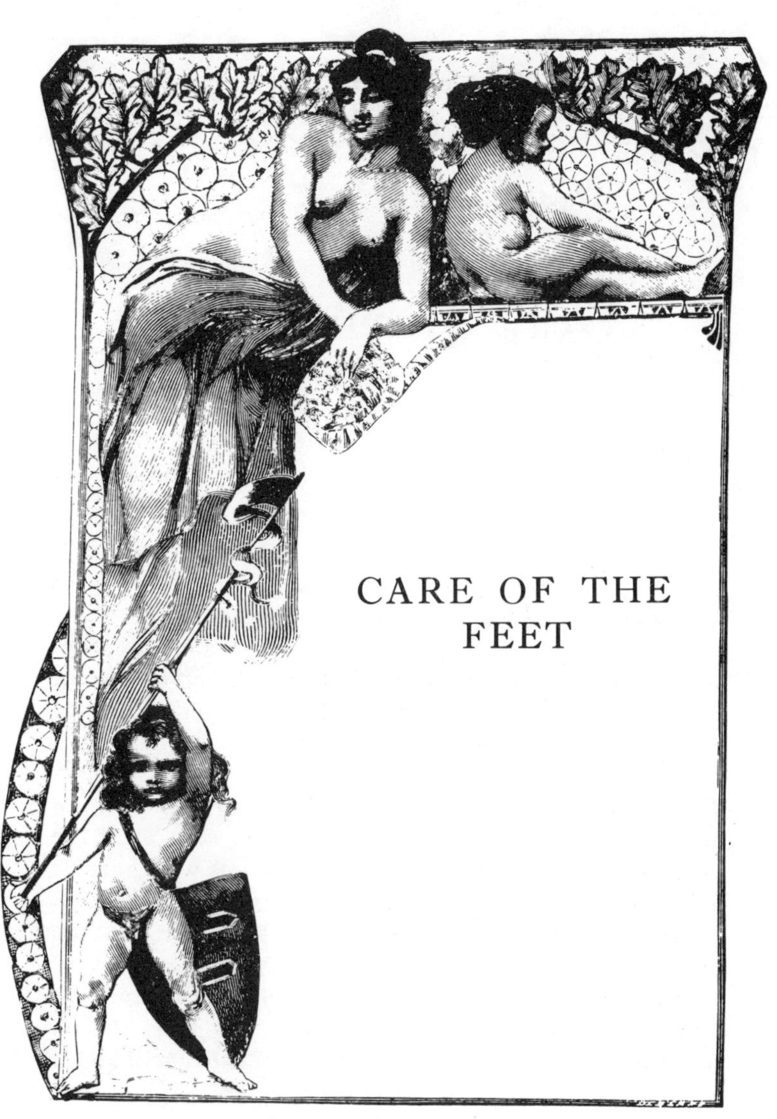

CARE OF THE
FEET

CARE OF THE FEET

EGULAR CARE of the feet is as important as regular care of the hands. The toe-nails should be kept well trimmed, but they should not be cut too short. Unlike the finger nails, they should be cut straight and not in a curve, as it is injurious to cut too far down into the side of the toe-nail. Doing this serves to increase the tendency of the nail to grow inwards at the corners where such a tendency exists. Boots with pointed toes should never be worn, as they compress the toes inwards in accordance with the shape of the boot, in some cases to such an extent that the great and little toes very nearly meet. The pointed shoe or boot is the cause of bunions, corns, and nearly every foot deformity. When corns and bunions make their appearance they should be at once treated, as, if neglected, they not only cause a large amount of pain, but in some cases nearly cripple the sufferer.

TO CURE INGROWING TOE-NAILS.

An ingrowing toe-nail can very often be cured in its first stages by the following simple means: With a sharp pair of scissors make a V-shaped incision in the centre of the top of the nail, and insert a piece of cotton wool between the nail and the toe at the corner in which the nail shows a tendency to grow into the flesh. The nail will gradually grow at each side towards the incision until the latter is closed, and the tendency to grow inwards at the corner of the toe will thus be effectively checked.

PERSPIRING FEET.

Some people are afflicted with feet that perspire to an abnormal degree. This is an extremely unpleasant affliction, arising very often from some defect in the general health. It frequently occurs in children, often disappearing altogether as they grow older; but with adults, as a rule, the trouble is more persistent.

In all cases strict cleanliness must be observed. The feet should be bathed at night in warm water to which a little Condy's Fluid has been added in the proportion of a teaspoonful of Condy's Fluid to a pint of water. They should be bathed in this way after any considerable exercise has been indulged in. Light woollen stockings should be worn—never cotton ones—and these should be frequently changed. Sometimes it will be found necessary to put on a fresh pair of stockings every day. Strict attention must also be given to the general health. In many cases it will be found that a good tonic will be beneficial.

There are some kinds of work which entail a woman being a great deal on her feet, and often her feet become very tired and sore in consequence. There is nothing more refreshing in these circumstances than to sponge the feet with a little methylated spirits. This treatment will cause the soreness and fatigue to disappear, and will, in addition, be wonderfully refreshing.

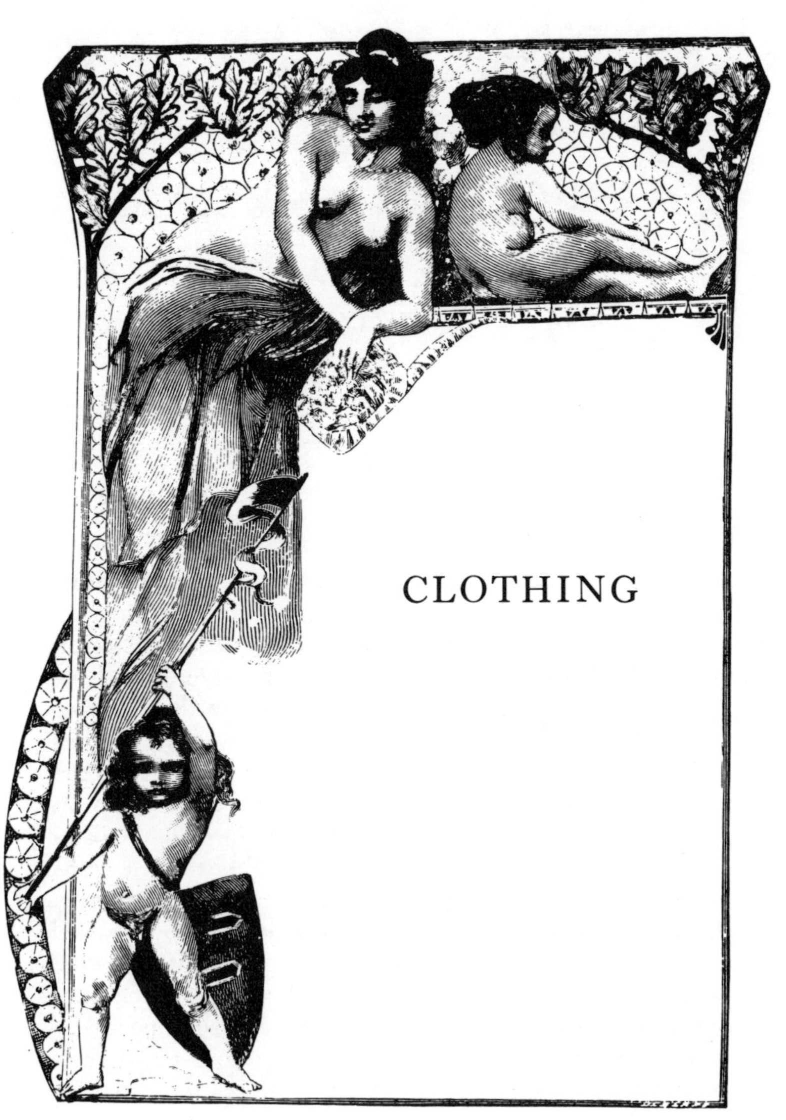

CLOTHING

CLOTHING

HE **PROPER** choice of suitable clothing for varying seasons forms an important factor in regard to our health. In winter the clothing should be light and warm—never heavy; in the summer it should be light and cool. All clothes should fit sufficiently loosely to give the limbs and respiratory organs their full freedom. In so far as protection against cold is concerned, woollen fabrics are superior to all other materials. Light woollen combinations or vests should be worn next to the skin in winter, and even in the summer, athletics, outdoor games, or any kind of violent exercise is indulged in, it is as well to wear a light woollen undervest, for wool is the only fabric which can be depended upon to absorb perspiration; and there is less risk of catching cold than when wearing linen or cotton next to the skin, as those fabrics become extremely damp after exercise, and very often a severe chill is the result. Colour should also play an important part in the selection of our clothing for the different seasons. For summer white is the ideal colour, as it is the one that absorbs the least heat. This is the reason why in tropical climates white is as much worn by men as by women. On the other hand, black or dark-coloured garments attract the sun and absorb the great amount of heat. These dark colours are ideal for winter wear, but they should not be much worn in summer.

BOOTS AND SHOES.

Suitable foot gear is a most important consideration. The question of fit is paramount. The boot must be made to fit the foot, and not the foot distorted out of all shape to fit the boot. Ill-fitting boots serve to deform the feet if their wear is persisted in, causing corns, bunions, enlarged joints, and ingrowing toe-nails and often other ills (see Care of the Feet).

Tight boots also impede the proper circulation of the blood, and chilblains in this way are often caused. The practice of wearing very high heels is particularly reprehensible. A woman wearing boots or shoes of this description cannot possibly walk in a natural fashion (see Exercise); the weight of the body is thrown forward upon the toes, being robbed of the support which the heels would have given it in the more natural circumstances; the heel of the shoe is placed in the middle of the foot under the arch of the instep—the result is to spoil and weaken the arch of the foot, and rob it of its natural spring; the gait becomes awkward, jerky, and ungainly in the extreme, and that freedom and swing of movement typical of a healthy and graceful carriage is conspicuous by its absence.

Well-cut boots and shoes with medium-sized heels and round toes are the ideal footwear. Very pointed toes are responsible for a great many of the toe deformities. It is not at all necessary that the footwear should be clumsy, it can be made just as neatly and as daintily with moderately sized heels as with high ones. They should have good strong soles, and not the thin brown-paper mixture which is so often characteristic of the cheap boot. It is a bad plan to economise in shoe leather—many a fatal chill has been traced to wet feet as a result of wearing poor shoes in inclement weather. In all cases where the soles of the boots or shoes are not waterproof, goloshes should be worn. Mothers should make their young daughters realise the importance of keeping their feet well protected from damp. Girls are apt to be very neglectful in this direction, and much ill health and even chronic invalidism in after life is very often the result.

THE CORSET.

Tight-lacing.—Few women realise how very injurious to their health this practice is. Tight-lacing has the effect of compressing the body to the point of deformity, and severe injury to the internal organs is often the result. Great care should be taken in the selection of corsets. It is wrong to economise in this direction. A little more money spent on the corset and a little less on dress and finery would have the effect of resulting in a much cleaner bill of health for many a woman who is accustomed to stint herself in this direction. Cheap corsets should never be worn; they are usually stiff, hard, and unyielding, not giving freedom to the movements of the body. The best corset-makers are now, however, building their corsets with more regard to the hygienic laws than was manifested years ago. Good corsets now are fairly elastic and

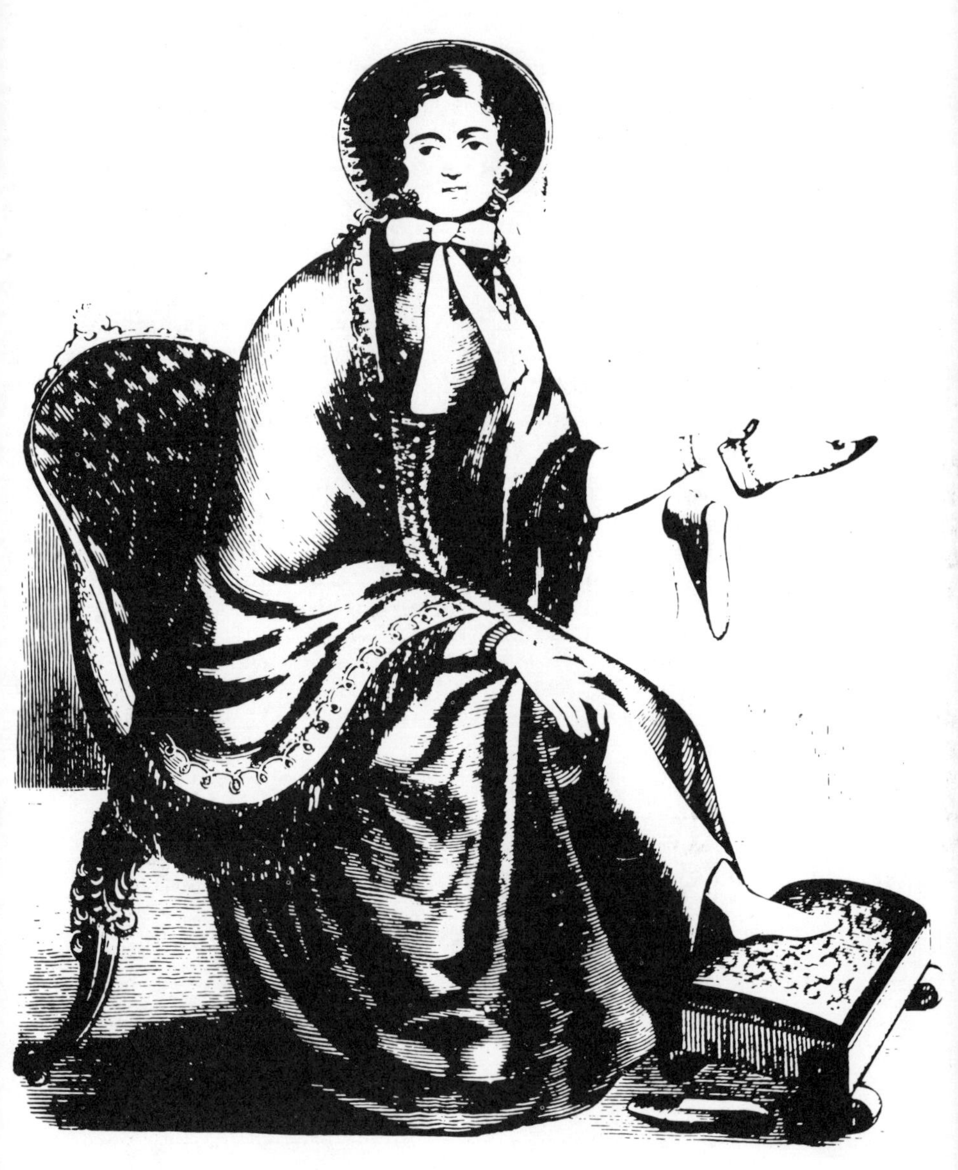

pliable. They are well planned and built, and are stocked in almost every size. It is always as well, if possible, to have the corset fitted, as this will ensure perfect ease in wear. Various makes are specially adapted for very full and very thin figures, and it is as well to bear this in mind when making a selection. Where the corset is fitted, the corsetiere will of course, adapt it to the special requirements of her customer.

It is as well to avoid the varying extremes of fashion in this direction. Though at one moment the "wasp" waist may be the decree, at another "no hips," slenderness almost to emaciation will be *de rigueur*, no woman who respects her health will become fashion's slave. By doing so she will often only succeed in making herself grotesque.

The sensible woman always knows how to strike the happy "medium" whatever the fashion may be; there is no more pleasing a sight than a good, well-proportioned figure well and sensibly corseted with due regard to the natural laws.

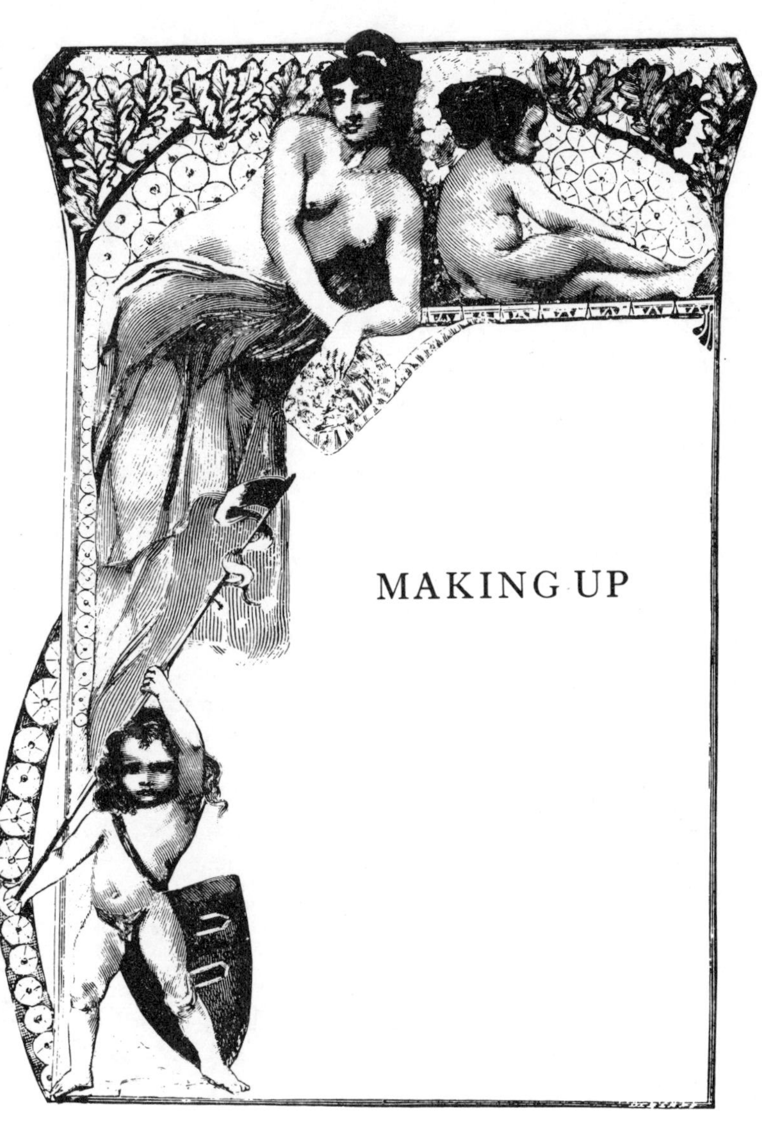

MAKING UP

MAKING UP

OW FAR it is justifiable to have recourse to art as an aid to good looks is, and has ever been, a much debated question. Before, however, trying to improve her appearance by the aid of "make up," a woman should pause and think, for once she has started making up there will be no going back; she will have to continue to do so. The pity of it is that it is most often the women whose skins and complexions leave nothing to be desired who are the first to have recourse to the aid of the rouge-box, and who thus inevitably ruin their natural complexions in the cult of the artificial.

There are some women, however, who, from chronic ill health or other causes, have such sallow, unpleasing-looking skins that one cannot blame them for seeking some sort of an aid to beauty—that is to say, if they make up so cleverly that the most practised eye cannot detect it. The art of make up lies in concealing the fact that art has been called in as an aid to nature. It is the clumsy and vulgar display of rouge, the emphasising of the fact that the complexion is false, that jars so much upon persons of refinement. On the other hand, one cannot help but admire the woman who makes up so cleverly that no one can tell her complexion is not natural.

The first care of the woman who makes up must be to do it well; secondly, and by no means less important, she must ever allow herself to be seen without her make up. She should make up the first thing in the morning, and not follow the example of some women who make a point of donning their complexions with their visiting toilettes. A woman who acts in this way cannot conceal the fact that she has recourse to art, as the difference between her natural complexion and her artificial one will be too marked to escape general notice.

HOW TO MAKE UP.

If a woman must make up it is necessary that she should know how to do so without injuring the texture of her skin in the process. Before attempting to apply the rouge, the face should be thoroughly washed with soap and warm water. After drying rub some good skin food well into the skin pores and wipe it off with a piece of rag. Then apply a small quantity of the rouge to the cheeks, finishing the process by dusting some good powder over the face. Take off all superfluous powder with a clean face chamois leather.

Rouge may be had in the form of liquid, powder, or paste.

Powder for the face is now in such general use that it has almost ceased to be regarded as a cosmetic. Yet in spite of this, great care must be taken in its application. The face thickly coated with powder is not pretty to look upon, and the pores of the skin become very much coarsened as a result of its indiscriminate use. Then some of the cheaper powders contain very injurious ingredients. Some face powders are, however, great boons to very greasy skins, but they must only be lightly dusted over the face with a clean powder puff or face leather, and then all superfluous powder should be dusted off. Care should be taken to use only the pure powders, avoiding all preparations containing mercury and arsenic. The Poudre Simon is one of the best face powders to be had. It should be used sparingly in conjunction with Creme Simon if possible. The Creme Simon, which is not the least bit greasy, should be gently massaged into the skin, and then rubbed off and the powder applied afterwards.

Care must be taken to remove all traces of powder and make up before retiring to rest at night. To do this some good. cold cream or white vaseline should be rubbed lightly over the face with a gentle massage movement, then wiped off with a piece of clean soft rag, and the face washed with soap and warm water.

The little leaflets known as Papiers Poudres are invaluable to the woman who is a great deal out of doors in the warm weather. They consist of diminutive sheets of paper finely powdered at one side and enclosed in a booklet form from which they are easily detachable. One of these little leaflets gently passed over the face when it is greasy and perspiring will remove not only superfluous moisture, but

all dust and dirt. The Papiers Poudres may be purchased
from most chemists.

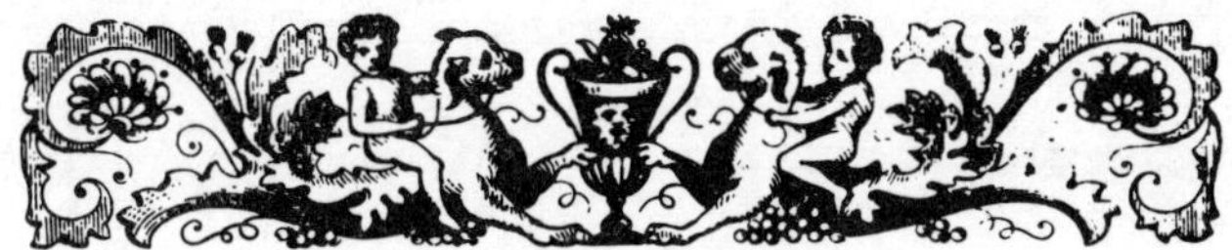

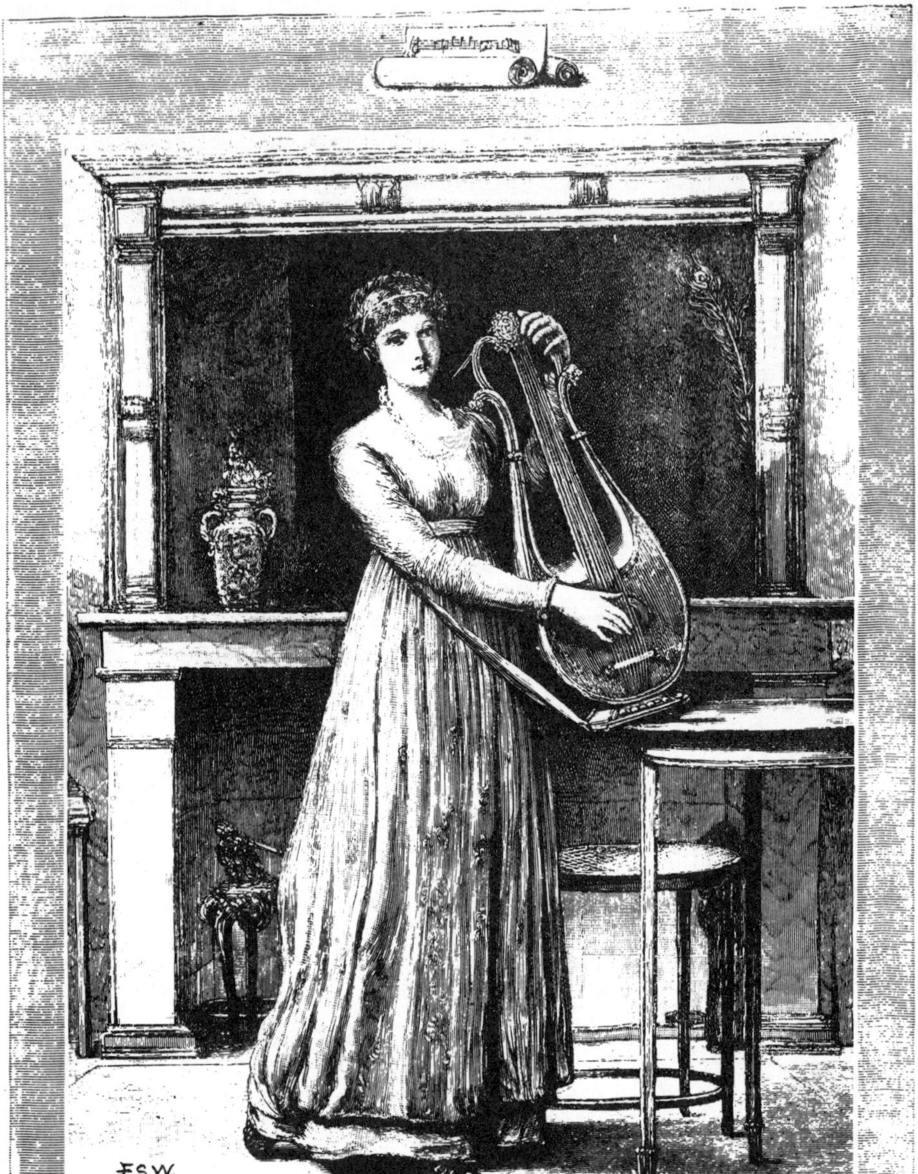

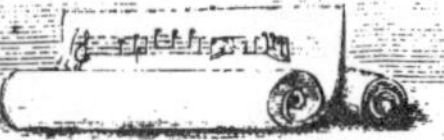

Music.
F.S.W.

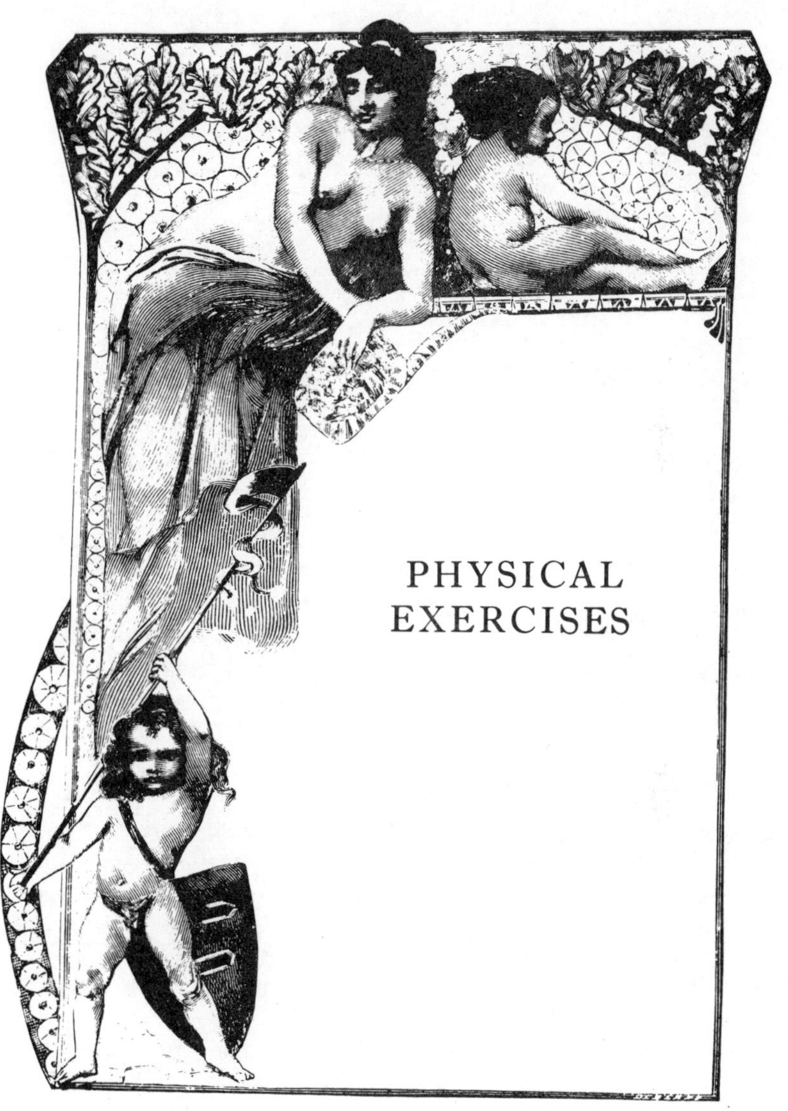

PHYSICAL EXERCISES

PHYSICAL EXERCISES

HE FOLLOWING simple physical exercises may be practised at home with much benefit. Any particular exercise or exercises may be selected and practised by a woman in accordance with her particular requirements.

First Exercise.—Position.—Stand with head erect and shoulders well squared, arms hanging at the side, the finger-tips touching the thighs, heels close together and toes turned out (Fig. 1).

Bend the forearms upwards, with the palms turned inwards and the fingers pointing to the shoulders (Fig. 2).

Throw out the arms sideways parallel with the shoulders, keeping the palms downwards (Fig. 3).

Second Exercise.—Stretch out arms sideways (Fig. 3)

then bend forearms until the hands are in front of the shoulders (Fig. 4). Then quickly stretch arms sideways.

Third Exercise.—Bend arms as in Fig. 2, then from this position stretch them forward, with the palms inward and the fingers well extended (Fig. 6).

The above exercises are especially good for chest development.

Fifth Exercise.—Stretch arms upwards (Fig. 5), then, with the feet firmly on the floor and without bending the knees, bend the body slowly backwards (Fig. 7). This exercise has most beneficial effects in strengthening the back. The beginner should take up her position at first near a wall against which she can support herself by her hands as she bends back.

Sixth Exercise.—Stretch the arms upwards (Fig. 5), then, without bending the knees, bend forwards until the tips of the fingers touch the floor in front (Fig. 8)..The knees must not be bent under any consideration. If you cannot touch the floor at first, bend as far as you can without bending the knees; the rest will come with practice. This exercise is of enormous value in giving suppleness to the figure, reducing obesity and strengthening the abdomen. It should be performed regularly by those who are inclined to stoutness. After practising Exercises 5 and 6 separately, practise both movements one after the other, bending backwards and forwards in turn several times.

Seventh Exercise.—Trunk-twisting movement. Place the hands behind the neck, the finger-tips just meeting (Fig. 9), twist the body slowly to the right (Fig. 19). Then after turning slowly to the front again, twist the body to

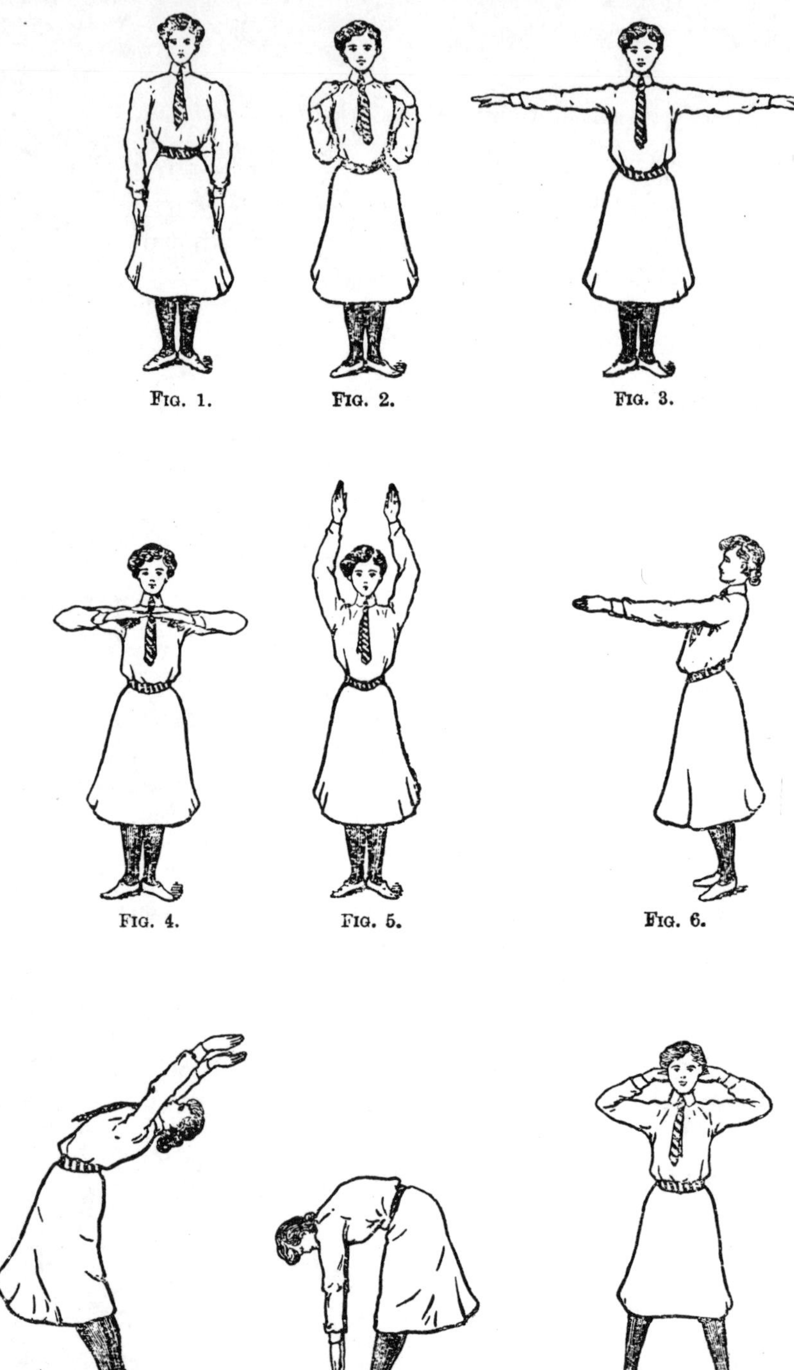

Fig. 1. Fig. 2. Fig. 3.

Fig. 4. Fig. 5. Fig. 6.

Fig. 7. Fig. 8. Fig. 9.

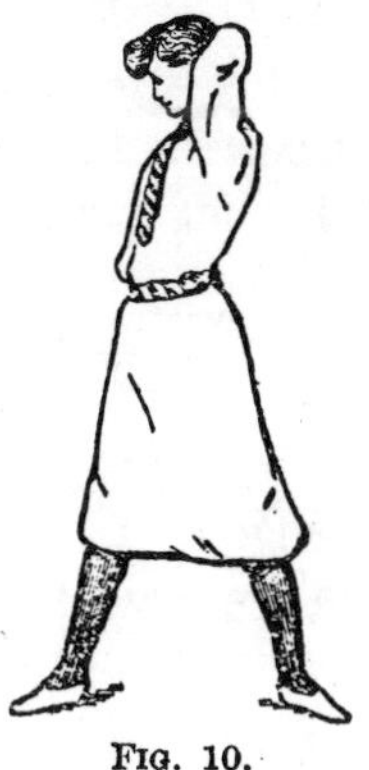

Fig. 10.

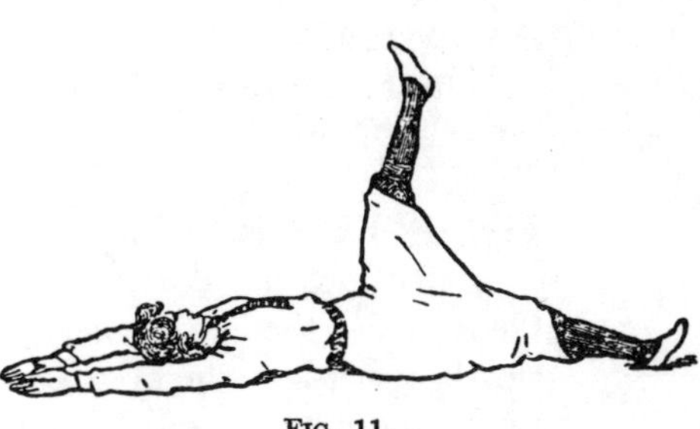

Fig. 11.

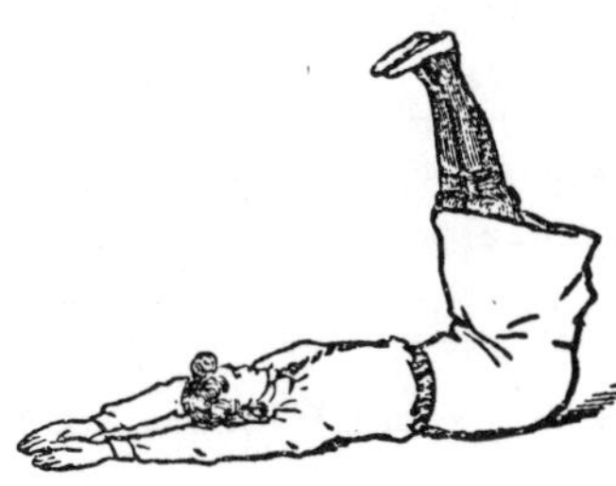

Fig. 12.

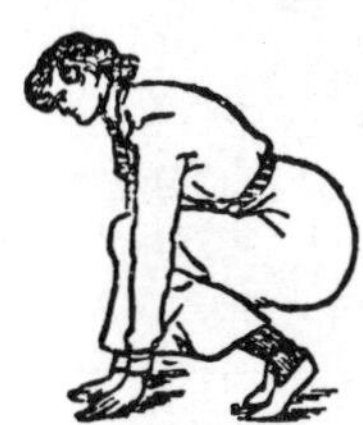

Fig. 13.

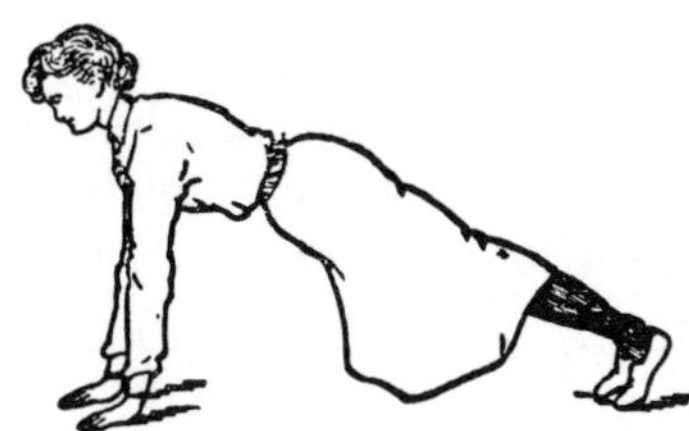

Fig. 14.

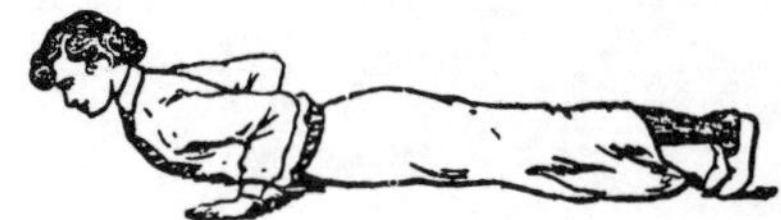

Fig. 15.

the left in the same manner. This exercise gives suppleness to the figure and has a most beneficial effect upon the internal organs.

Eighth Exercise.—Lie down on the floor with arms extended behind the head and the feet well together. Gently raise the left leg as high as it will go (Fig. 11), then slowly lower it to the floor again. Raise and lower the right leg in the same manner. Repeat several times, then raise and lower both legs together (Fig. 12). This is also an effective exercise for reducing superfluous flesh and curing constipation and digestive troubles.

Ninth Exercise.—Bend the knees as in Fig. 13, placing both hands on the ground in front of you. Then, without bending the arms, throw out the legs to the rear (Fig. 14). Bend the arms until the chest nearly touches the floor (Fig. 15). Then straighten the arms until the position is again the same as Fig. 14. Return to position shown in Fig. 13.

This exercise is also very good for digestive troubles.

THE VALUE OF HOUSEWORK.

Housework is a source of exercise which has a decidedly health-giving value. Turning mattresses and making beds are very ordinary and seemingly uninteresting household duties, but from the point of view of health they are good; the more energy and interest a woman displays in following the ordinary routine of her domestic duties, the less danger does she run of becoming a victim to nerves and other kindred feminine complaints. She must not overdo things, however, as it is as harmful to work too hard as to work too little, but if she goes through with her light household duties cheerfully and willingly, taking pleasure in her work, they cannot but be productive of physical benefit to her. It is not everyone who can indulge in tennis, golf, and other similar outdoor and health-giving exercises, but there are very few women who have an excuse for not availing themselves of the exercise to be had in the daily routine of household work. Let them therefore, if they value their health, make the most of their opportunities in this direction.

BREATHING.

Few women have realised the value of deep breathing as an incentive to vitality and health; fewer still know how to breathe correctly. In breathing the lips should be kept closed and the breath inhaled and exhaled through the nostrils. Six to ten deep breaths taken regularly every morning upon rising will act as a wonderful tonic to the system. Standing erect with the hands upon the hips, inhale a deep full breath whilst slowly rising upon the tips of the toes—then slowly exhale whilst bringing the heels to the ground again. This breathing exercise should be repeated at least six times every morning or evening, and the number of breaths could be gradually increased to ten or twelve with the utmost benefit. Through the day-time, when working, walking, or indulging in any kind of exercise, a woman should practise the art of breathing correctly, inhaling and exhaling the breath through her nostrils and not through her mouth, as is the habit with many.

WALKING.

To walk gracefully, the body must be erect, but not stiff, and the head held up in such a posture that the eyes are directed forward. The tendency of untaught walkers is to look towards the ground near the feet; and some persons appear always as if admiring their shoe-ties. The eyes should not thus be cast downward, neither should the chest bend forward to throw out the back, making what are termed round shoulders; on the contrary, the body should be held erect, as if the person to whom it belongs were not afraid to look the world in the face, and the chest by all means be allowed to expand. At the same time, everything like strutting or pomposity must be carefully avoided. An easy, form, and erect posture is alone desirable. In walking, it is necessary to bear in mind that the locomotion is to be performed entirely by the legs. Awkward persons rock from side to side, helping forward each leg alternately by advancing the haunches. This is not only ungraceful but fatiguing. Let the legs alone advance, bearing up the body.

UTILITY OF SINGING.

It has been asserted, and we believe with some truth, that singing is a corrective of the too common tendency to pulmonic complaints. Dr. Thrush, the eminent physician, observes on this subject: "The Germans are seldom afflicted with consumption; and this, I believe, is in part occasioned by the strength which their lungs acquire by exercising them in vocal music, for this constitutes an essential branch of their education. The music master of an academy has furnished me with a remark still more in favour of this opinion. He informed me that he had known several instances of persons who were strongly disposed to consumption, who were restored to health by the exercise of their lungs in singing."

THE WEATHER AND THE BLOOD.

In dry, sultry weather the heat ought to be counteracted by means of a cooling diet. To this purpose cucum-

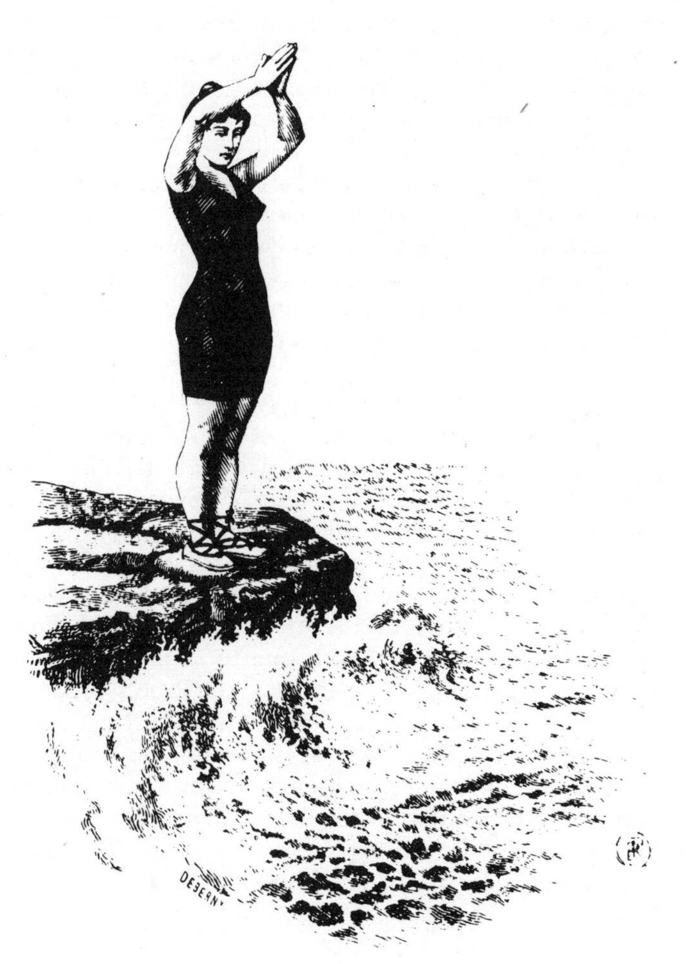

bers, melons, and juicy fruits are subservient. We ought to give the preference to such alimentary substances as lead to contract the juices which are too much expanded by the heat, and this property is possessed by all acid food and drink. To this class belong all sorts of salad, lemons, oranges, pomegranates sliced and sprinkled with sugar, for the acid of this fruit is not so apt to derange the stomach as that of lemons; also cherries and strawberries, curds turned with lemon acid or cream of tartar; cream of tartar dissolved in water; lemonade, and Rhenish or Moselle wine mixed with water.

HOW TO GET SLEEP.

How to get sleep is to many persons a matter of high importance. Nervous persons who are troubled with wakefulness and excitability usually have a strong tendency of blood on the brain, with cold extremities. The pressure of the blood on the brain keeps it in a stimulated or wakeful state, and the pulsations in the head are often painful. Let such rise and chafe the body and extremities with a brush or towel, or rub smartly with the hands, to promote circulation, and withdraw the excessive amount of blood from the brain, and they will fall asleep in a few moments. A cold bath, or a sponge bath and rubbing, or a good run, or a rapid walk in the open air, or going up and down stairs a few times just before retiring, will aid in equalising circulation and promoting sleep. These rules are simple, and easy of application in all cases.

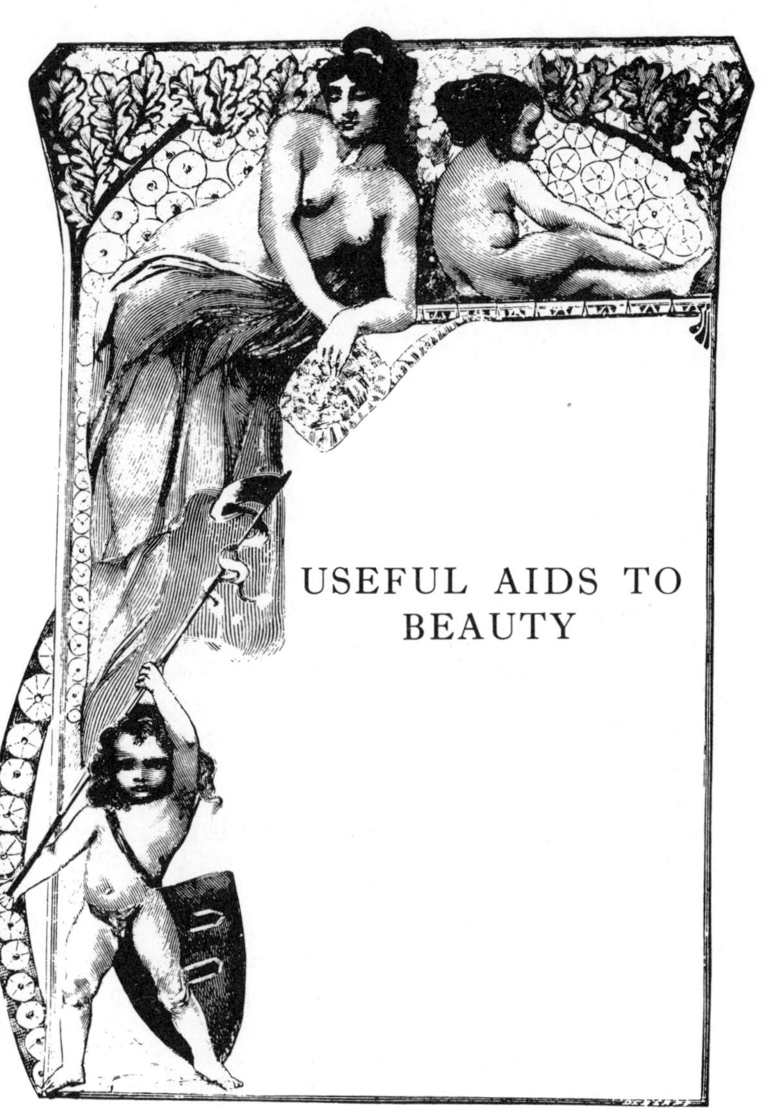

USEFUL AIDS TO BEAUTY

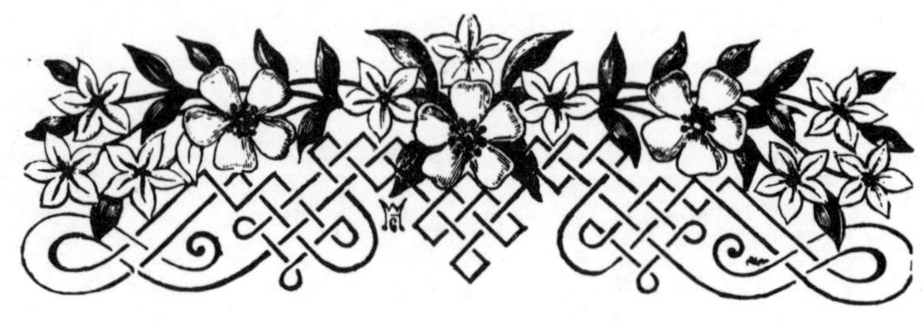

USEFUL AIDS TO BEAUTY

A VERY PLEASANT PERFUME.

ALSO A preventive against moths, may be made of the following ingredients: Take of cloves, caraway seeds, nutmeg, mace, cinnamon, and Tonquin beans, of each one ounce; then add as much Florentine orris root as will equal the other ingredients put together. Grind the whole well to powder, and then put it in little bags among your clothes, &c.

LAVENDER SCENT BAG.

Take of lavender flowers, free from stalk, half a pound; dried thyme and mint, of each half an ounce; ground cloves and caraways, of each a quarter of an ounce, common salt, dried, one ounce, mix the whole well together, and put the product into silk or cambric bags. In this way it will perfume the drawers and linen very nicely.

LAVENDER WATER.

Essence of musk, four drachms; essence of ambergris, four drachms; oil of cinnamon, ten drops; English lavender, six drachms; oil of geranium, two drachms; spirit of wine, twenty ounces. Mix all together well.

HONEY WATER.

Rectified spirit, eight ounces; oil of cloves, oil of bergamot, oil of lavender, of each half a drachm; musk, three grains; yellow sanders shavings, four drachms. Let it stand for eight days, then add two ounces each of orange-flower water and rose water.

HONEY SOAP.

Cut thin two pounds of yellow soap into a double saucepan, occasionally stirring it till it is melted, which will be in a few minutes if the water is kept boiling around it, then add a quarter of a pound of palm oil, a quarter of a pound of honey, threepennyworth of true oil of cinnamon; let all boil together another six or eight minutes; pour out and let it stand till next day, it is then fit for immediate use. If made as directed it will be found to be a very superior soap.

THE HANDS.

Take a wine glassful of eau-de-Cologne, and another of lemon juice; then scrape two cakes of brown Windsor soap to a powder, and mix well in a mould. When hard, it will be an excellent soap for whitening the hands.

TO WHITEN THE NAILS.

Diluted sulphuric acid, two drachms; tincture of myrrh, one drachm; spring water, four ounces, mix. First cleanse with white soap, and then dip the fingers into the mixture.

A delicate hand is one of the chief points of beauty; and these applications are really effective.

STAINS.

Stains may be removed from the hands by washing them in a small quantity of oil of vitriol and cold water without soap. Salts of lemon is also efficacious in removing ink-stains from the hands as well as from linen.

COLD CREAM.

1. Oil of almonds, one pound; white wax, four ounces. Melt together gently in an earthen vessel and when nearly cold stir in gradually twelve ounces of rosewater.
2. White wax and spermaceti, of each half an ounce; oil of almonds, four ounces; orange-flower water, two ounces. Mix and directed for No. 1.

TO SOFTEN THE SKIN AND IMPROVE
THE COMPLEXION.

If flowers of sulphur be mixed in a little milk, and after standing an hour or two, the milk (without disturbing the sulphur) be rubbed into the skin, it will keep it soft and make the complexion clear. It is to be used before washing. The mixture, it must be borne in mind, will not keep. A little should be prepared overnight with evening milk, and used the next morning, but not afterwards. About a wineglassful made for each occasion will suffice.

EYELASHES.

To increase the length and strength of the eyelashes, simply clip the ends with a pair of scissors about once a month. In eastern countries mothers perform the operation on their children, both male and female, when they are mere infants, watching the opportunity whilst they sleep. The practice never fails to produce the desired effect.

88

Dissolve two ounces of borax in three pints of water; before quite cold, add thereto one teaspoonful of tincture of myrrh, and one tablespoonful of spirits of camphor; bottle the mixture for use. One wine glassful of the solution, added to half a pint of tepid water, is sufficient for each application. This solution, applied daily, preserves and beautifies the teeth, extirpates tartarous adhesion, produces a pearl-like whiteness, arrests decay, and induces a healthy action in the gums.

CAMPHORATED DENTIFRICE.

Prepared chalk, one pound; camphor, one or two drachms. The camphor must be finely powdered by moistening it with a little spirit of wine, and intimately mixing it with the chalk.

MYRRH DENTIFRICE.

Powdered cuttlefish, one pound; powdered myrrh, two ounces.

AMERICAN TOOTH POWDER.

Coral, cuttlefish bone, dragon's blood, of each eight drachms; burnt alum and red sanders, of each four drachms; orris root, eight drachms; cloves and cinnamon, of each half a drachm; vanilla, eleven grains; rosewood, half a drachm; rose-pink, eight drachms. All to be finely powdered and mixed.

QUININE TOOTH POWDER.

Rose pink, two drachms; precipitated chalk, twelve drachms; carbonate of magnesia, one drachm; quinine (sulphate), six grains. All to be well mixed together.

HAIR DYE.

To make good hair dye some lime must be first obtained, and reduced to powder by throwing a little water upon it.

The lime must then be mixed with litharge in the proportion of three parts of lime to one of litharge. This mixture, when sifted through a fine hair sieve forms the most effectual hair dye that has yet been discovered.

Directions for Application.
Put a quantity of the mixture in a saucer, pour boiling water upon it, and mix it up with a knife like thick mustard; divide the hair into thin layers with a comb, and plaster the mixture thickly into the layers to the roots, and all over the hair. When it is completely covered with it, lay over it a covering of damp blue or brown paper, then bind over it, closely, a handkerchief, then put on a night-cap, over all, and go to bed; in the morning brush out the powder, wash thoroughly with soap and warm water, then dry, curl, oil, &c. Hair thus managed will be a permanent and beautiful black.

Hair Dye, usually styled Colombian, Argentine, &c., &c.
Solution No. 1. Hydrosulphuret of ammonia, one ounce; solution of potash, three drachms; distilled or rain water, one ounce (all by measure). Mix, and put into small bottles, labelling No. 1.
Solution No. 2. Nitrate of silver, one drachm; distilled or rain water, two ounces. Dissolve and label No. 2.

Direction for Application.
The solution No. 1 is first applied to the hair with a tooth brush, and the application continued for fifteen or twenty minutes. The solution No. 2 is then brushed over, a comb being used to separate the hairs, and allow the liquid to come in contact with every part. Care must be taken that the liquid does not touch the skin, as the solution No. 2 produces a permanent dark stain on all substances with which it comes in contact. If the shade is not sufficiently

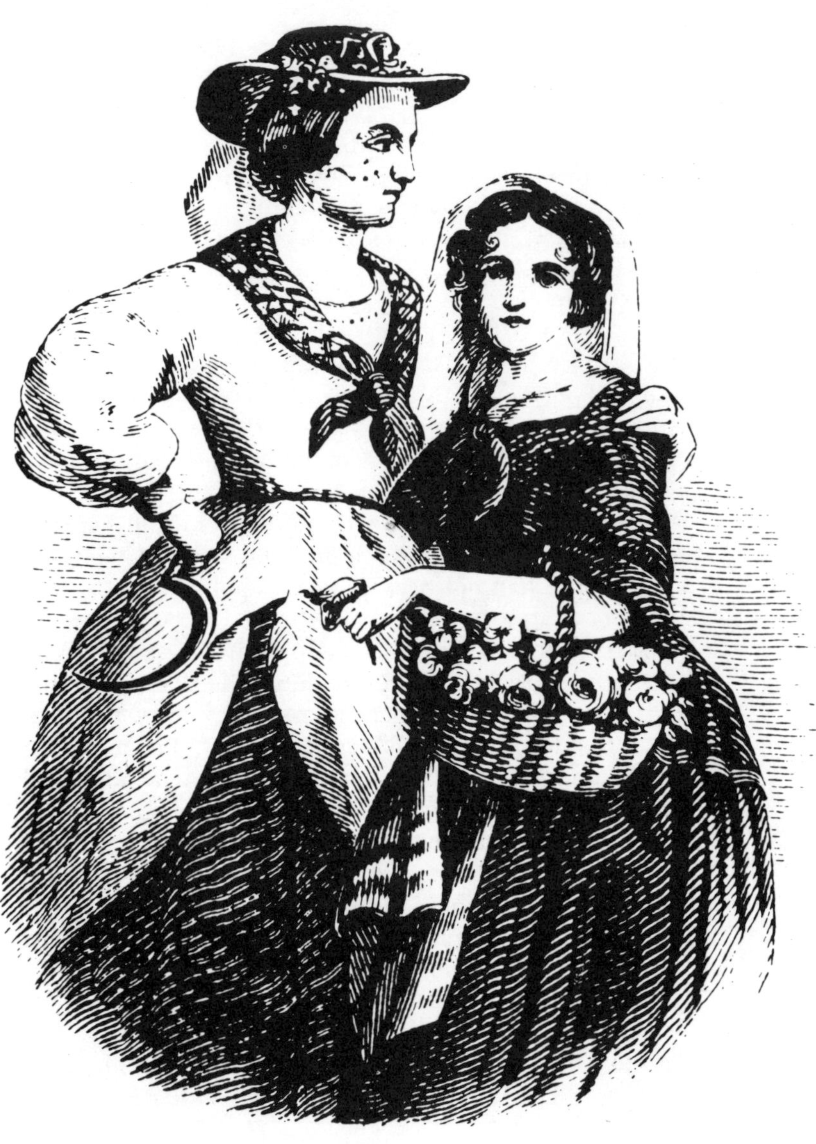

deep, the operation may be repeated. The hair should be cleansed from grease before using the dye.

TO TEST HAIR DYE.

To try the effect of hair dye upon hair of any colour, cut off a lock and apply the dye thoroughly as directed above. This will be a guarantee of success, or will at least guard against failure.

THE PROPER APPLICATION OF HAIR DYES.

The efficacy of hair dyes depends as much upon their proper application as upon their chemical composition. If not evenly and patiently applied, they give rise to a mottled and dirty condition of the hair. A lady, for instance, attempted to use the lime and litharge dye, and was horrified on the following morning to find her hair spotted red and black, almost like the skin of a leopard. The mixture had not been properly applied.

COMPOUNDS TO PROMOTE THE GROWTH OF HAIR.

When the hair falls off, from diminished action of the scalp, preparations of cantarides often prove useful; they are sold under various high-sounding titles. The following directions are as good as any of the.more complicated recipes.

POMADE AGAINST BALDNESS.

Beef marrow, soaked in several waters, melted and strained, half a pound; tincture of cantharides (made by soaking for a week, one drachm of powdered cantharides in one ounce of proof spirit), one ounce; oil of bergamot, twelve drops.

ERAMUS WILSON'S LOTION AGAINST BALDNESS.

Eau-de-Cologne, two ounces; tincture of cantharides, two drachms; oil of lavender or rosemary, of either ten drops.

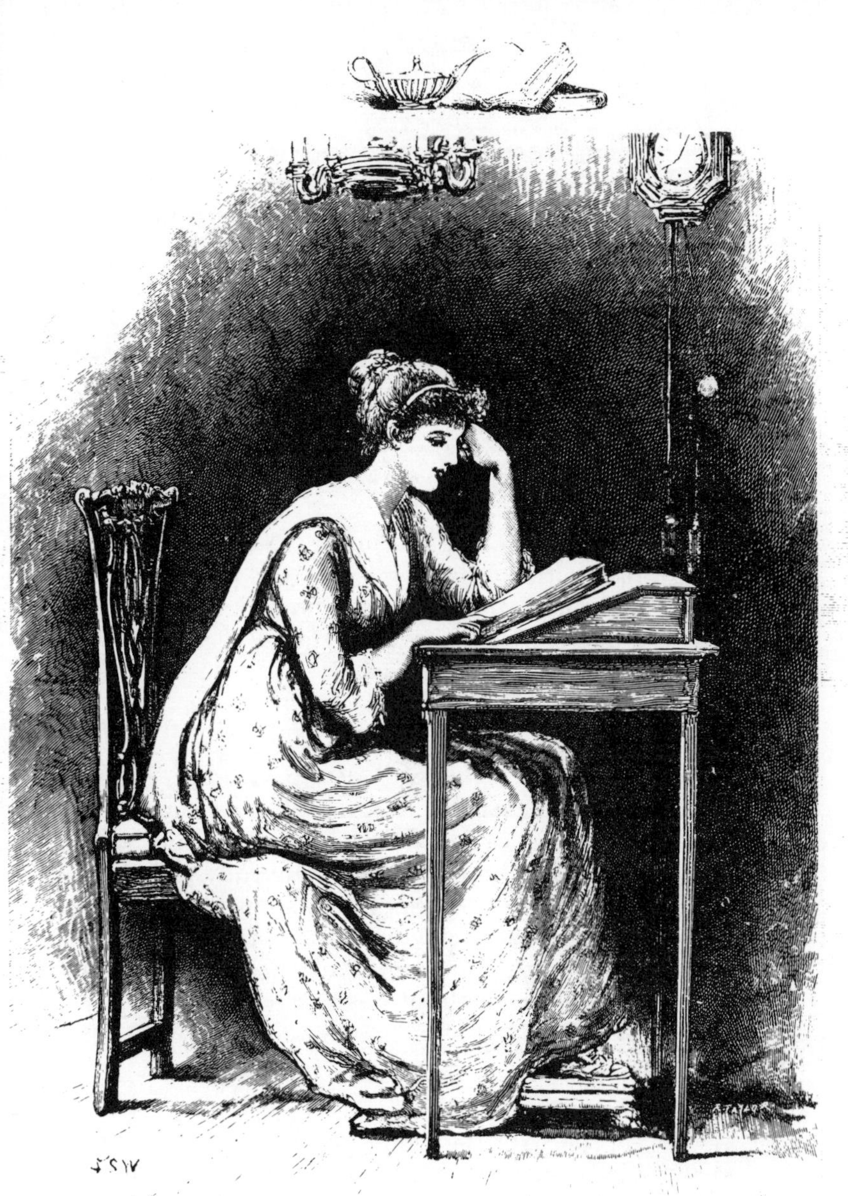

Literature

The applications must be used once or twice a day for a considerable time; but if the scalp becomes sore, they must be discontinued for a time, or used at longer intervals.

BANDOLINE OR FIXATURE.

Several preparations are used; the following are the best:
1. Mucilage of clean picked Irish moss, made by boiling a quarter of an ounce of the moss in a quart of water until sufficiently thick, rectified spirit in the proportion of a tea-spoonful to each bottle, to prevent its being mildewed. The quantity of spirit varies according to the time it requires to be kept.
2. Gum tragacanth, one drachm and a half; water, half a pint; proof spirit (made by mixing equal parts of rectified spirit and water), three ounces; otto of roses, ten drops; soak for twenty-four hours and strain. Bergamot may be substituted for otto of roses.

EXCELLENT HAIR WASH.

Take one ounce of borax, half an ounce of camphor; powder these ingredients fine, and dissolve them in one quart of boiling water; when cool, the solution will be ready for use; damp the hair frequently. This wash effectually cleanses, beautifies, and strengthens the hair, preserves the colour and prevents early baldness. The camphor will form into lumps after being dissolved, but the water will be sufficiently impregnated.

HAIR OILS.
Rose Oil.

Olive oil, one pint; otto of rose, five to sixteen drops. Essence of bergamot, being much cheaper, is commonly used instead of the more expensive otto of roses.

Red Rose Oil.

The same. The oil coloured before scenting, by steeping in it one drachm of alkanet root, with a gentle heat, until the desired tint is produced.

POMATUMS.

For making pomatums, the lard, fat, suet, or marrow used must be carefully prepared by being melted with as gentle a heat as possible, skimmed, strained, and cleared from the dregs which are deposited on standing.

Common Pomatum.

Mutton suet, prepared as above, one pound; lard, three pounds; carefully melted together, and stirred constantly as it cools, two ounces of bergamot being added.

Hard Pomatum.

Lard and mutton suet carefully prepared, of each one pound; white wax, four ounces; essence of bergamot, one ounce.

CASTOR OIL POMADE.

Castor oil, four ounces; prepared lard, two ounces; white wax, two drachms; bergamot, two drachms; oil of lavender, twenty drops. Melt the fat together, and on cooling add the scents, and stir till cold.

SUPERFLUOUS HAIR.

Any remedy is doubtful; many of those commonly used

are dangerous. The safest plan is as follows: The hairs should be perseveringly plucked up by the roots, and the skin, having been washed twice a day with warm soft water, without soap, should be treated with the following wash, commonly called MILK OF ROSES: Beat four ounces of sweet almonds in a mortar, and add half an ounce of white sugar during the process; reduce the whole to a paste by pounding; then add, in small quantities at a time, eight ounces of rose water. The emulsion thus formed should be strained through a fine cloth, and the residue again pounded, while the strained fluid should be bottled in a large stoppered vial. To the pasty mass in the mortar add half an ounce of sugar, and eight ounces of rose water, and strain again. This process must be repeated three times. To the thirty-two ounces of fluid, add twenty grains of the bichloride of mercury, dissolved in two ounces of alcohol, and shake the mixture for five minutes. The fluid should be applied with a towel immediately after washing, and the skin gently rubbed with a dry cloth, till perfectly dry. Wilson, in his work on Healthy Skin, writes as follows: "Substances are sold by the perfumers called depilatories, which are represented as having the power of removing hair. But the hair is not destroyed by these means, the root and that part of the shaft implanted within the skin still remain, and are ready to shoot up with increased vigour as soon as the depilatory is withdrawn. The effect of the depilatory is the same, in this respect, as that of a razor, and the latter is, unquestionable, the better remedy. It must not, however, be imagined that depilatories are negative remedies, and that, if they do no permanent good, they are, at least, harmless; that is not the fact; they are violent irritants, and require to be used with the utmost caution."